# Through the Pain

## The silent suffering of a Personal Trainer

## by

## John K Frazier

# Prologue

As I sit down to write this book, I realized I don't know how to write. I mean I know how to write but not a book. Being dyslexic (which is a really hard work to spell for someone with dyslexia) writing a book does not seem the most fun you will ever have. Also, when I started to write this book, I thought I was writing a fitness book but a few chapters in I realized that It's a motivational book (I hope). Which means I had to go back and re-write some of it. I started by writing only things that seem to relate to my fitness life. But I realized that my life hasn't been just about fitness. My whole career I have been a personal trainer, I added massage therapy about seven years into that. But I have also been an actor the whole time too. In fact, I started my own personal training business (Frazier Fitness) when I was 22 years old. That was in order to have the time to audition, which is what actors do, a lot. More of that to come.  I have something to say, and no one can say it for me. So here it goes.

Why "Through the Pain"?  The purpose for the title is to describe my life, my story. I was diagnosed with Ankylosing

Spondylitis when I was 27 years old. Oh, Ankylosing Spondylitis or A.S. for short is an arthritic condition that attacks the spine and hips and can ultimately lead to fusion of the spine. Real fun stuff. We'll get more into that later.

I've been a personal trainer for the past 30 years, so that's where "The Silent Suffering" came from. Because literally I suffered for years and didn't talk about it. But why write about it? Good question. I think I have grown tired of people thinking that because you're a trainer, they think that you have to look perfect. Especially now that I'm an older trainer and that my disease is progressing, I don't have a perfect body. I know shocker, right. I mean, I'm alright. But Trainers are people too! They get hurt have aches and pains, don't always eat right, get tired, don't want to exercise sometimes, get depressed, and God forbid gain and lose weight.  But it does happen because we are actual people. For far too long I feel like personal trainers have been put up to a weird high standard. Trainers come in all shapes and sizes. If you met a female trainer who was 5'5 and 180 lbs. you might not think much of her as a trainer. But if you found out that she was 325 lbs. two years ago, you would ask where I can sign up. Just because a guy has a six pack doesn't mean he can or knows how to get you one. I'm going to hold back from a six pack of beer joke here. Way overdone in the fitness community.

So, I think you see where I'm heading with this book. "Don't judge a book by its cover". I also, hope to part some sort of wisdom here in this book.  Maybe teach people that staying healthy, and fit doesn't always mean having the best body.

Or the fact that obstacles can be overcome but we know that from "Rocky" So maybe you will just learn not to put personal trainers on a pedestal. Or maybe you'll just laugh and cry and enjoy a story.  Or maybe you won't get anything out of it, I don't know, I haven't written it yet. Seems like I'm off to an O.K. start. Despite all the misspellings (and I just misspelled misspelling) and the fact that I have no idea what I'm going to write next, not bad.

I'm going to tell you a story, my story. The good, the bad and everything in between. O.K., maybe not everything, just stuff that pertains to the story.  Hopefully you'll laugh, you'll cry, you'll pass a watermelon. But I know one thing; it will be truthful, thoughtful, and very easy to read because I don't know a lot of big words. I've read this in a book before, so I'll use it now, "Let's begin."

# Chapter One

## The Beginning

As every story goes there is a beginning. Mine starts as a child, as early as I can remember having physical problems.  Now not all my physical problems have to do with A.S. Some are just life stuff and others, well are just hard to believe happens to just one person. Put your feet up and let's begin.

 I was five years old when my first injury happened. We were on our way to school. My mom was driving and me and my two sisters were sitting in the back. My mom was driving a 1969 Ford LTD. A big car, like a tank. The back seat was one long bench and I was sitting behind the driver's seat. As my mom dropped us off, we had to exit the right side of the car because the left side was the street side. My oldest sister exited the car follow by my other sister. Now I was little at the time so I had to crawl across the bench to exit the car. So, as I'm crawling out and almost to the door my sister without looking slammed the door behind her. You've heard of getting your finger caught in the car door, well try your head. That's right my head was slammed in the car door. Now first I want to note that I don't blame my sister in anyway. She was only six and had no idea that I was coming out that door. Even though that was 47 years ago, I still remember how painful that was. Obviously, I had a concussion but back then you didn't go to the doctor unless you were almost dead. My sister felt bad and I did get out of school for the day. But man, did I have one big headache.

What's more ridiculous than getting your head slammed into a car door? Getting you head slammed in a car door a second time. Yes, a month later the same thing happened again. I couldn't help but to blame my sister a little bit. Still, love ya sis. And that started it off, the luck of the Irish, but not in a good way.

Over the next years I will befall many weird accidents and injuries. Obviously, this has little to do with being a personal trainer, but it sets the background that leads to that decision.

The next main injury I remember has to do with a lawn mower. As a child I always worked. My dad and mom worked hard and provided for us but there wasn't a lot of extras to go around. So, to buy the toys I wanted or to go to the movies or later when I wanted "cool clothes" to wear, not just the stuff my mom would buy at Kmart, I would work. My first job was mowing lawns. I started in fifth grade mowing my parents' yard then the next-door neighbor then the lady down the street and eventually I almost had the entire circle. Yes, we lived on a circle street. Now one wet day when I was in sixth grade, I had to cut the next-door neighbor's yard. I grew up in Garland Texas, a suburb of Dallas. And in the summer, we would get a fair amount of rain. Biblical whether we like to call it in the south. It had been raining for a few weeks in early summer so I couldn't mow any lawns. With all the rain the grass grew fast and thick which means when I could get to mowing it was going to be very difficult. You see, back in the 1970's we didn't have power mowers. Well, if they did, we didn't. I used my dad's push mower with a pull start cord. With the grass really high and still wet I had to kind of get a running start to hack at the grass. I would hit the tall grass for a few inches and then get stuck and have to back up and take another running start. So, this would happen row after row and to make matters worse the bag would fill up very quickly. I was having to unload the bag into a trash bag almost after every row. To make matters even worst I would have to keep the motor running on the mower because if I shut it off it might not start again. I would however slow the mower down when I took the bag off. Thank God I did that, or I might not be writing this book. Halfway through when I took the bag off, I noticed that a lot of wet grass had built up on the opening from the mower to the bag, which was making it hard for the grass to go into the bag. In my hast I decided to clean the wet grass from the opening knowing full well that the mower was on. I got most of the grass that was blocking the opening when I slipped. Did I mention that the grass was wet? In one second the blade of the mower split my middle finger twice. Now that hurt A LOT!

Bleeding a lot, I ran inside of my house where my mom started screaming. I was sick and felt like I was going to pass out. My dad came into the room and calmly counted my fingers. I remember him counting, one, two, three, and then He got to ten, so everything was there. Time to go to the hospital. This injury would surely need stitches, right. No, the doctor decided to just butterfly it and it would be fine. It took somewhere between three to four months to close up and made it hard to play guitar, which I did at the time. Now that I think about it, that's probably why I was never good at playing guitar. Or maybe I just sucked but I'm going to blame the accident.  I did heal and still have the scar to this day. Told you there wouldn't be a dull moment. And it only gets worse from here.

Now seventh grade the worse thing I can remember is tackling a guy at football practice and his shoulder pad went right through my facemask and cut me right between the eyes to the bone. It didn't hurt much but I knew I was bleeding, so I ask the coach how bad was it and he almost passed out, so I knew it was bad. Again, I don't know why but I didn't get stitches and it took a while to close up. Especially because every time I put my helmet on it would open up a little. It also left a scare but this one is more obvious because well it's between my eyes. The only way to cover it is to grow a unibrow. On to eighth grade where I suffered my biggest injury so far. Yes, football. I was a running back in grade school and quit a good one, but it didn't start that way. I'm the only boy of four children and I have two older sisters and one younger. I didn't rough house with brothers like others, so I didn't have a reference to be tough. The first practice in seventh grade was very intimidating. We did the one-on-one tackle drill where one guy carries the ball between two cones with another guy about four feet away. So basically, it's just head-to-head hitting. Mono e mono. Naturally, the coach puts me up against the largest guy on the team. I'm 127 lbs. soaking wet, and the guy seemed like he was 300 lbs. Of course, he was probably only 190 but still that is a lot of difference. I got crushed. Pancaked, I think they call it. The coach got in my face and said that's the hardest hit you're going to take. He was wrong of course but I didn't die, so that was something. My dad watched the whole practice since it was the first practice. I could tell that my dad was disappointed. He probably was thinking that his kid is a wimp and he's going to get killed. He tried to teach me about intensity so when we got home, we went one on one. Me in pads and my dad not in pads. I remember thinking that I was going to hurt him. I still wasn't getting it. I didn't want to hurt anybody. But without intensity I was going to get hurt. So, my dad did the only thing he could think of to show me intensity. He kept saying you have to tense up like you are going through a brick wall, like the side of the house. He got halfway across the yard and ran as fast as he could and put his shoulder into the side of the house as hard as he could. I don't know if you have ever seen a man run full speed at a brick house (I know I never had before or since) but as soon as he hit the house, it made him fly back several feet doing a backwards summersault in the air and somehow land on his feet. And then he yells, "that's how you do it".  My mother ran out of the house screaming, "it's an earthquake, it's an earthquake." (We live in Texas) That's how hard he hit the house. The next day my dad tried to hide it, but he was in tons of pain. It looked as if he couldn't raise his arm and didn't for a week or two, but he wouldn't lead on that he was hurt. I know what you are thinking, but every word of that story is true. I know it's not about my pain but it's too good of a story to leave out. And yes, I did learn about intensity.

Fast forward to my eighth-grade year where I'm a very good running back. I had speed but I could also run over guys. This one game I broke outside and was running down the field.

About fifty yards down the field a guy had the angle on me and caught me. But I wouldn't go down easily. He slowed me down enough to have about five of his teammates catch me and started jumping on my back. I'm at the twenty-yard line and I really want to score a touchdown but the weight on my back was too much, and I started to go down. On the way to the ground, I put my right hand out and when I did it, my arm got caught on the ground. As I hit the ground the weight of all the guys pushed me forward, but my hand stayed in the ground making my fingers go all the way back to my forearm. It hurt so bad. I got up screaming and no one knew why. The coaches gave me attitude like I was wimping out, which really pissed me off. So, I wrap an ace bandage around it and went back into the game. I don't remember the rest of the game because I was in so much pain, but I did play. I ended up in a soft cast because I tore every tendon and ligament in my wrist. But I put a pad over my cast and never missed a game. I believe that was the start of me learning how to be tough and able to take pain. Which was probably good because there was a lot more in my future.  A lot more. Now the last thing I remember from grade school is my knees. Between fifth and sixth grade I grew a lot. Fifth grade I was short and pudgy. By sixth grade I probably grew six inches. I was tall and thin but with one problem Osgood-Schlatter disease. Now it's known as Osgood-Schlatter condition which is "a painful condition characterized by tiny micro fractures of the bony bump in the lower leg bone where the ligament from the kneecap is inserted into the lower leg. The bump is known as the tibia tubercle. It is a disorder of the early teens, especially during a growth spurt, more likely to affect young men than young women, especially athletes of either sex who are active in games requiring substantial running and or jumping." Thanks WebMD. I played basketball so check, check that, and oh yeah, check again. I fit everything in that statement. But I didn't know that it would hurt for so many years. From sixth grade through most of high school. It was mostly O.K. but if I fell on my knees, OMG what pain that was. I started playing basketball with knee pads which helped a lot, but it always hurt some. What, "stop you say". That's silly I love playing basketball, so through the pain I go. For the rest of my grade school years, I don't remember any more major injuries. I'm sure there were minor injuries along the way, but nothing compared to the ones I mentioned. Now sit back and relax because here comes high school. Not a dull moment there.

## Chapter Two

## High School Years

Clean slate is what I was thinking. Some people from eighth grade went on to the same high school and I had one good friend, but I wanted to break out of my shell. You see, even though I was an athlete in grade school I wasn't considered cool by any means. I was shy and a little closed off. I remember being very awkward then, but I realize now that everybody was awkward at that age. I remember being very excited to meet new people and I wanted to be very out-going. So, I talked to everybody. I knew some people from other schools because I had played sports against them in grade school. But when you play football, you have immediate friends. I could hit and take a hit and I didn't say much so I was cool. Now injuries did not occur my freshman year. Other than little aches and pains I didn't seem to have anything major but that's when my back started to hurt. Very tight, muscle spasms on the lower left side but nothing I couldn't handle. I played football, basketball, and ran track. Also, I was in the musical and on student counsel. Now the musicals are where I found the girls. Guys were so dumb when they thought that the musicals were stupid. It was where the girls were. Lots and lots of girls. Senior girls, too! Which doesn't hurt when you're a freshman. I got to be friends with senior girls during the musical "Bye Bye, Birdie" They would pass notes to me in the hall between classes and came up to me and gave me kisses on the cheek. Guys in my class were amazed. By the way, I know this doesn't have anything to do with my story about injuries but it's still a great story and had a lot to do with my confidence. That year was a turning point on how I would turn out. It's funny the things you look back on and realized how it shaped your life. The confidence I gained in my freshman year changed the course of my high school career and started to shape who I'd become. I played sports because I loved to play them but by doing so, I guess it made me "popular", I just didn't know I was.

My freshman year was also important because I took a speech class. Still, I was a little shy, but this class would bring me out of my shell. Kit Sawyer was my teacher and with her help I was slowing gaining confidence. I remember one presentation where I dressed up like Richard Simmons and did my presentation. If you don't know who he is, you can go to YouTube and find out. That will give you an idea how much I was coming out of my shell. It was the first time I remember getting genuine laughs. That made a big impact on me. I also got an A which was rare. Remember dyslexia. (Spell check again, still can't spell that word.) Anyway, my teacher asked me to try out for the play. As mentioned, we were doing "Bye Bye Birdie" a very fun musical. We did a musical every year but for some reason we always called it a play. Are you in the play? Going to play practice. Which is fitting because it was a lot of fun, and we were playing. I decided to try out even though I really couldn't sing. Little did I know, if you were a guy, you were probably going to make it. In fact, I think everybody made it that tried out, it was just to decide what role. So of course, I made it as chorus. No real part just background. But I was interacting with girls in the upper classes. Heaven for a freshman. Shortly, into rehearsals the guy playing Birdie had to drop out and one of the guitar guys moved up to play Birdie. So, there was a part that was open. To this day I don't know why they gave me that part. Did they see something in me, did they want to bring me out of my shell? I don't quit know but it was probably a pivotal point for me to be an actor today. Thanks Kit and Joe. The girls in the play had to act as if we were super famous (Birdie was like Elvis) so they would scream and paw at us because I was part of the band. Now in the TV version there are no guitar men but in our version there was. And thank God there were.

So, the pretend bleed over to real life which is why senior girls passed notes to me and gave me kisses. This gave me confidence and broke me out of my shell. So, I guess you could say that's when the acting bug hit me and hit me hard.

Now going into my sophomore year, the routine was the same. Football "two a day" in the Texas heat of August.  Now my next injury came two weeks into the season during practice. A junior player let's call him Shane, because that was his name. He thought I was stepping out with his girl, so he was unhappy with me. The truth is I was just friends with "his girl". I was friends with a lot of girls in high school. Anyway, I played defensive end and Shane was a wide receiver on offensive. He came in motion and when the ball was snapped, he did a crack-back block on me. Which is a blind block because I'm facing toward the quarterback. Now I'll never know what exactly happened and what he hit me with, but it was either a fist or elbow. He hit me under the facemask right on the chin. And yes, it knocked me completely out. I woke up and all I could see was green, so I thought I was facing down but in fact I was on my back facing up. I thought that he had knocked the colors out of me. He didn't and I started to see colors again shortly after. Knowing what I know now things would have been handled differently. Back then no one thought much of concussions as they do today. It was more shake it off and keep going so that's what I did. That concussion was on Monday, and we played our next game on Thursday. The hits I took or gave out gave me another concussion, but I was so out of it that I played the whole game and then collapsed after the game. I don't remember the game at all. This time though I would go to the hospital and was diagnosed with a concussion and would miss the next few weeks. I don't know if any of you have had a concussion, but it does make you feel bad for weeks. Headaches of course but tired, nauseous, and generally feeling pretty shitty.

I wish I could tell you that that was the only concussions I got in my life but that would be a lie. I estimate that I had at least 12 concussions in high school. Most concussions, I never told anybody for fear of not playing. (I know how dumb that sounds now but in high school especially in Texas, football was life.) I wanted to get a football scholarship to college and then play for the Dallas Cowboys. That was the plan.

So there where many games that I would be knocked senseless, and the trainer would put smelling sauce under my nose and then back in the game. I know, I know, that sounds bad. It sounds bad to me and I'm writing this. Thank God that today they know so much more and take it more seriously then back then. Now you are wondering what ever came of all those concussions. Well, as an adult I have had two head CT's and there were no long-term drain bamage, I mean brain damage. I have learned a lot about concussions and damage to the brain over the years and I have wondered if my depression has been a side effect of the concussions. Depression is a huge factor when one is talking about head trauma. I don't know if I will ever know for sure but it probably had an effect on it. I just don't know to what extent. Speaking of depression don't worry there's a whole chapter about it later on. Next up, the back.

I remember my back started hurting my sophomore year. Doctors said growing pains, muscle weakness, muscle spasms, or whatever. The logical thing for the doctor was to give me a back brace and muscle relaxants and let it rip. Worse idea ever. It felt better to wear the back brace so I would sometimes wear it to school and always when I played football. And no high school kid should be taking muscle relaxants all the time but I was. Maybe not every day but more than I should. But what did I know? I know now that wearing a back brace was the worst thing I could have done because by wearing the brace all the time I weakened the muscles which made it worse. A back brace should only be used when you are doing something that could hurt your back. i.e., Moving furniture, heavy boxes, lifting heavy weights, or if your back is in really bad shape and the only way to get around is to use a brace. When I have a flare up of A.S. I wear my back brace to train clients but I take it off when I'm not training them. I'm sure you have seen the guy in the gym that wears a huge weight belt the entire time they workout.

Well, that is the wrong thing to do. You want your muscles to do most of the work. Only use a weight belt if you are doing heavy squats or dead lifts. Which most people should not be doing. (I know that is going to piss some people off in the fitness industry but unless you are a body builder or professional athlete, you can do more harm than good, lifting heavy weights.)  "Core" has been the word that the fitness industry has been using for years. But that is exactly what you want to use while exercising.

So throughout high school I wore a back brace and took muscle relaxants which only made things worse and lead to other injuries. Looking back on it, it's so obvious that I had Ankylosing Spondylitis but it would still be another ten years before the diagnoses. Definitely, should not have power lifted my senior year. It made my back so much worse but I was tough, I could take it. The thing that I didn't know was that my pain was not usual. I thought everybody hurt that much. When they said suck it up, I did. I didn't know that your bones weren't supposed to hurt that much.  And the leg pains I would get and still get was and is so painful. That is from the arthritis swelling and pinching the nerves in my back giving me pain and throbbing in the bones in my legs. Most the time it is only in one leg and on the rare _fun_ occasion it's in both. This pain can bring me to tears and re-think wanting to be alive. It can also get to the point where my leg will have a hard time working. I kind of start dragging my leg. Pain meds, Ibuprofen, and rest, is the only thing that helps. Luckily, it usually only lasts one day and the longest it lasted is four days.

Most of my sophomore year was uneventful. Normal high school stuff. Lots of angst insecurity and general confusion. I was considered "popular". I didn't really think about it. I remember really wanting to be liked. Not popular, just wanted to be liked. I don't know why really. I think to some degree we all just want to be liked, even if we don't admit it. We want to connect. It's part of the human condition. We are not meant to be isolated. Now don't get me wrong I love my alone time. But it's mainly just to recharge my battery. Some of us do just fine with a hand full of friends. But in high school I wanted to be everybody's friend. Most people reading this

would think that I was a jerk. Football player, "popular" must be a jerk. But I wasn't. I talked to everybody. Even if I didn't hang out with someone outside of school, didn't mean I wasn't nice to them. I went out with my friends that I spent the most time with and they happen to play football as well. But when you spend as much time with the same group of guys, you're bound to forge some friendships. Not all the football players were nice to everybody. Some acted like you would think. Some of the things I would hear about, that they did were pretty bad but I was never there when they did bad stuff. I was very busy in high school. I played all the sports and I was in student counsel, the musicals, and I also worked on the weekends. Thinking back on it I don't know how I did it all. I was tired all the time.  I was very driven and just never stopped. Now, I have to slow down and conserve my energy. I can't do half the stuff I use to be able to do. But back then it was go, go, go.

Sophomore year we did the musical "Mame" This was probably my least favorite of the musicals we did. I was only a good enough singer to be in the chorus, again. No big part like my freshman year. So maybe a little let down. I would try to make the most of the bit parts they would give me. In "Mame" for some reason there was a flasher in one scene. I don't remember why but it was a quick bit. I had a trench coat on and my back was to the audience so I just had on a tee shirt and shorts under. One performance, as kids would do, we thought it would be funny if I didn't have anything on under the trench coat. I was way too shy to go without any clothes so I decided to wear my tidy whities, which is funny enough, and enough to throw off the main actress. My friend also drew on my chest a smiley face and an arrow pointing down to my tidy whities. I was nervous to do the stunt and, in my nervousness, I forgot to do one really important thing. Unbuttoned the bottom button on my trench coat. I'm supposed to enter stage right stand in front of the main actress and quickly open my coat. With the bottom button buttoned my trench coat didn't open all the way. The actress still got to see the goods but so did everybody in the wings (the sides of the stage that the audience can't see.) Not only that but the audience got a peek of my butt through my tidy whities. It was quick but it was out there. I did make the main actress laugh but one of my teachers in the wings was not amused. Well, maybe a little. I can't believe that I didn't get in trouble for it. In fact, I never got in trouble even though I did a few things I should have gotten in trouble for, but the teachers liked me. I never did anything really bad just being a kid. I knew early on to make friends with the teachers. Even if

I didn't like them; they would never know. They were the gate keepers If I wanted to play sports, I had to pass my classes. School was hard for me. I only caught maybe half of what was being taught. I could only do half the reading they would assign each night. At the time I didn't know I was dyslexic. For a long time, I thought I just wasn't smart. In grade school there was a time when I thought I was "retarded". Mainly because a girl called me that. I know something was really wrong because I couldn't do the work other kids were doing. It got to the point that my parents held me back in the fourth grade. A very hard thing for a kid to have to go through. I didn't understand it at the time but my parents did the best to make it OK. They asked if there was anything I wanted to do and I said Karate. So, for a few years I took Karate at the YMCA. Even being held back, school was still very hard for me. I remember always having a tutor in grade school. But when I went to high school there was no time for a tutor. Most teachers would be available after school and I went to them quite often. I "acted" interested in the school work, and "acted" like I really wanted to understand the material. To me it was just a means to an end. I lived for the extra stuff in high school and the book stuff was the pathway to that. I'm convinced that I was given some passing grades because I acted like I really cared. Probably some of my best acting to this day.

The rest of sophomore year was pretty uneventful. Played football, basketball, and ran track. During football season I started out on the JV team. Mostly made up of sophomores and some juniors that didn't make the varsity team. But some juniors played JV and varsity. As a small sophomore pulling guard there was no way I would make the varsity team, at least that's what I thought. Now the varsity and JV teams practice separately but on the same field. One day at practice we were going through hitting drills. My friend Chris and I were hard hitters, so they would usually put us up against each other in straight one-on-one hitting drills. It was basically "kill each other". Chris stood at least 4 inches taller than me and probably at least 70 lbs. heavier, maybe more. We were friends (and still are to this day) but we would have epic battles at practice. No animosity, just good competition.  This day was another epic battle. But this time it caught the ears of the head coach of the varsity team. I say ears because he was on the other side of the field and only could hear Chris and me battling. We hit each other so hard that it made a very loud cracking sound that could be heard 100 yards away. After the drill, we went back to the end of the line so we could go again. I was seeing stars and was very wobbly. Little did I know Chris was feeling the same way. He leaned over and asked me if I could see. I said not too well. We slowly started to lean on each other to hold ourselves up. As we were trying not to pass out, the head coach of the varsity came over and said "what the hell was that". Our coach said it was us and he called us over to practice with the varsity. So now I'm playing varsity and Junior varsity. JV played on Thursday nights and varsity played on Friday nights of course. I started both ways on JV and I probably wouldn't see any playing time on varsity. Just a backup on the sidelines, just in case. I guess you know where this is heading. And yes, on the first game I suited up the starter got hurt at the beginning of the game so I played most the game. I did well from what I remember but it must have been funny to see me as a starting offensive lineman. That year I was probably all of 150 lbs. soaking wet. Most of the defensive lineman for the other teams were at least 200 lbs.

but more like 220-240. I couldn't go up top on these big guys so I would just aim for their knees. Mostly got a hold of their ankles but wouldn't let go. I'm sure it looked like a Chikwawa nipping at the heels of a grow man. It mostly worked because all I had to do is get myself between the defender and the running back and tie up the defender for just a few seconds. I'm not going to say I was successful every time but more times than not, I was. That year we were bad, really bad. I don't remember how many games we won but it wasn't many. When one of your "big men" on the line was me you probably not going to win too many games.

My junior year was similar to my sophomore year. I still played football, basketball and ran track. I was in the musical and student council. The only major injury was the ongoing concussions which I had every year playing football. I can't remember how many I had each year, but as I mentioned probably 12 total throughout high school.

The musical we did was probably the best one we did in all four years I was there. "West Side Story"! It was a really hard musical to do. The dance numbers were epic and we tried to do them exactly like they were done in the movie version. We worked really hard and created a very good musical, especially on the high school level. Again, I didn't have a big part because I wasn't a strong singer. But I still enjoyed doing the musicals and wanted to do the best job I could. I wasn't thinking at the time about a career in acting. I was still thinking about a professional football career. That would change my senior year.

Going into my senior year of high school I was determined to be in the best shape of my life and get a football scholarship to college. Enter a graduate from my high school who was working out at our high school gym. He was massive and looked like he knew what he was doing. He took me under his wing and worked out with me every day. Now I haven't said this yet but I was very naive back then and really didn't know anything. One day "my workout partner" wanted me to take a supplement but I would have to inject it. I didn't know at the time that he meant steroids but I was like " I don't know about that." I don't think at the time that I even knew what steroids were. I told him I would have to talk to my coach, so we did. "My workout partner" went with me to ask my coach if I could take his supplement. What balls this guy had. (Or didn't if you know what steroids does to you.) My coach seemed as naive as I was and said he didn't think it would be a good idea. Thank God that he did, otherwise I might have taken them and I would have had even more problems than I already do. I continued to work out hard making small gains putting on maybe ten pounds. Now other guys were making huge gains of 25 to 50 pounds of muscle. Yeah, you guess it, "my workout partner" was supplying  guys with steroids. I guess I was working out with a drug dealer, who knew. I surely didn't. Like I said; naive. Now, this is where the story takes an unexpected turn.

Football Two-a-days start in August. For the whole summer I had been working out for about 3-4 hours a day. Weights, running, football drills, you name it I was doing it. I even did an exercise that the coach would only use for punishment; air-raids. That's when you run full speed on the football field and when the coach blows the whistle you dive to the ground, immediately push yourself back up and continue running. With no coach I would just tell myself to dive down. I think I was a little nuts. Most people need someone to motivate them to push themselves pass the point they can push themselves but I was different. It all paid off. My resting heart rate was 43. Yes, I know that's really low. The doctor took my pulse and started to laugh. I asked what was wrong, and he said nothing, other than most people would be asleep with that low of a resting heart rate. I was ready for the football season to start. Two-a-days started and it wasn't very challenging to me. Other guys were throwing up and I was running circles around them. In fact, one day after practice, I stayed on the field and ran extra sprints because practice wasn't hard enough. The coach saw this and yelled at me to get in the locker room and get showered. I realize later although he was impressed with me and he just wanted to get home to his wife and child. After breezing through two-a-days my senior year started. This was going to be my year. I lived and breathed football and I was going to dominate.

The time has come! The week of our first game. It's a Tuesday morning and I wake up very tired. It wasn't that unusual because of football and school starting and all the other activities I was involved in, I was tired all the time in high school. As the day when on I could barely keep my eyes open. I think I sleep through every class that day. Seventh period rolls around which for me was athletes, which means football. We would lift weights until after school when the rest of the football team got out of school and then practice would start. I go to seventh period and then tell the assistant coach that I was feeling really, really bad.  He said I could lay down in the trainer's room and sleep until practice started. I put on my football pads and passed out on the trainer's table. Next thing you know I'm being woken up by the head coach who was pissed. (Side note: the other coaches knew me and knew I was the hardest working guy they had.) What I lacked in skill I made up in heart. I wasn't the fastest, strongest, biggest player but I was the toughest. The head coach was new and didn't know me. I was one of the leaders on the team. I would motivate the other guys and pick them up when they were down. This is why I think the assistant coach let me sleep because I never complained. The head coach not knowing this was pissed. He grabbed me and through me out the door to go to practice. And I did. Now I'm not lying when I tell you I don't remember the practice. My body went through the motions and I don't know if anyone knew how sick I was. I know I was running fever but that was it. Next thing you know I'm sitting on the floor of the locker room and I remember asking a few of my teammates to help me take off my pads. When they did, they jumped back almost like they had seen a ghost. Well, I was pail but also had a really back rash all over my body. I probably looked like I had the Ebola virus. They started screaming for the coach to come in and when he saw me, he turned white as a ghost. Knowing that he made me practice, probably scared the shit out of him. By this point I couldn't do anything. I knew I couldn't drive and one of my teammates drove me home. At first, I think they thought I had the measles or mumps or something like that. I don't remember how it went down but I do know that I sleep for 48 hours straight. Only waking up for my mother to give me sips of water. I was so weak that I couldn't get out of bed. Probably should have been in the hospital. I don't remember going to the doctor but I was diagnosed with mono. A really bad case. Although I was heart-broken that I wasn't going to be able to play in the first game, I was just so sick that I couldn't even be that upset about it. Friday rolls around, and it's game day. For the brief minute that I was awake, I asked my dad if he could go to the game and tape it for me. He did and came home to show me the game. He woke me and I was too weak to walk to the couch, so he picked me up and carried me to the couch. Which was a big deal because my dad was 5'6 maybe 150 and I was 5'10 165. He laid me down and started the game and I immediately fell asleep. I saw parts of the game and we won, but I wanted to be out there. This probably was the first real disappointment in my life. At first it was hard to even care because I was so sick. But as the next week came, I started to feel better. I wanted to get back to school. The sooner I started back to school the sooner I would be able to play football. That's what I thought. What I didn't know was how serious my illness really was. At some point I read a story about a quarterback at another school in the same area that had gotten mono during two-a-days that same summer. Fatigue was his complaint but during the August heat in Texas, every football player had fatigue. He got hit during practice and his spleen ruptured and he died. The spleen filters the blood and when you have mono the spleen doubles or triples in size. Normally the spleen is protected by the rib cage but when it swells it is exposed. Had I taken a hit that day at practice, I wouldn't be writing this story.  Which leads me back to the story. I wanted to go back to school that next week but the doctor said that if I got bumped in the hallway my spleen could ruptured. Probably couldn't have gone that week anyway because I think I slept the entire week. The next week I was feeling better but still wasn't allowed to go to school. I missed two and a half weeks of school before I was allowed to go back. Now missing two and a half weeks of school at the beginning of my senior year was not easy to catch up on. In fact, I don't know how I did catch up. I think the teachers just felt sorry for me and just passed me. By this time, I had missed two football games and the only thing I was thinking was getting back to playing. I knew I needed to catch up on schoolwork so I started there. I wasn't allowed to exercise at all, plus just going to school wiped me out. After the second week at school my dad and I made a plan to eat really healthy and start to exercise, even though I couldn't go to football practice. I rode my bike and lifted weights. Now I was weak. Very weak. I had lost 20 pounds and since I had no body fat back then, it was all muscle. I went to work to get myself back into shape so when the doctor cleared me, I could go right back to playing. I ate a lot, sleep a lot and did my school work. Every week my dad would pick me up from school and take me to the doctor to check my blood count. When you're sick your white blood cells go way up. I think mine went as high as 80,000 and normal is around 10,000. Until my white blood cells went down to 10,000, I couldn't play. Week after week I would go to the doctor and he wouldn't clear me. Then I would take a doctor's note to my football coach and he would be upset. Not nearly as upset as I was. I got very depressed. I thought my world was ending because I couldn't play football. Silly now but when you are in high school everything is the end of the world. That might have been the first time I had to deal with depression. I have battled depression my whole life but I think that was the first time I can remember being depressed. I'll talk about depression in a later chapter.

All my hopes and dreams were in football. I wanted to get a scholarship to play football in college because I knew that would be the only way I could go to college. My grades weren't good enough to get a scholarship so football was it. Plus, I really loved playing the game.

There are ten games in the season and with each week that went by, my hopes of playing were fading. By now we have played six games. I once again went with my dad to the doctor on that Monday. But this time he said that I was clear to start exercising again. We didn't tell the doctor that I had already been working out for weeks.  We took the, "cleared to exercise" that I could play football. I mean football is exercise. Now the ride back to school was very exciting, knowing that now I was going to be able to go to practice. Practice was already in progress. My dad and I went to the locker room, went to my locker for the first time, grab my helmet and shoulder pads (Monday practice was in shorts, not full pads) and ran out to the field. As I got to the field guys started to realize that I was coming to play and they started clapping. Everybody was happy to see me return. My dad followed me to practice and pulled the coach a side. Now I couldn't really hear what my dad said to him but my dad was pointing his finger and looked really intense. I did hear my coach say a few times "yes sir, yes Mr. Frazier". I could guess what my dad was saying, something to the effect of you better make sure my son is O.K. The funny thing is, my dad is all of 5'6 and 150 lbs. and my coach was 6'1 probably 240. And my dad was looking up at my coach shaking his finger. It was like a mouse taking on a cat and winning. But soon the excitement would fade into reality that I no longer had my starting position. Great, I'm back on the team but I'm not going to play. Way back in 'two a day" the coach said anyone could challenge another player for a starting position. You would go one on one. So, either that first day or the second day of practice I told the coach I wanted to challenge for my starting position. At the time I weighted 165 lbs. and played guard on the offensive guard. When I came back, I only weighted 150 lbs. Either weight is too small to be playing on the offensive line but we were a small school and most guys were the size of a running back which is what I use to play.  During a break in practice the coach called the guy that took over my position and me to the field to go one-on-one. I had a big chip on my shoulder for missing the first six games of the season. I kind of wanted to destroy the poor guy. And I think I did. I was very weak at the time but I still handled the guy. Now the coach was put in a tough position because nobody had ever taken him up on "the challenge". He decided to let him play the first half and me the second. I wasn't happy with that but I had a chance. Also, I was back-up defensive end and linebacker. I could have started on defense but the coach tried to have guys only started on offense or defense. I thought I would try to get in the game any way I could. It had been a long and painful process to not play the sport that I loved. I had hopes of not only playing in college but to get a scholarship. At this point I knew that was probably not going to happen. All I wanted to do is play the best four games I could possibly play. I worked so hard to get back on the playing field, not just physically but with all the make-up homework.  School was hard enough but being dyslexic (I didn't know at the time) and two weeks behind was damn near impossible. I somehow got all my grades up except for one. The teacher failed me. My parents and the school got involved and the teacher let me take the test over again. This time I passed and was able to play in the game.

Game day. I was nervous because I knew I was still very weak. I was still very tired and would fall asleep in class or anywhere actually. But my determination and heart were bigger than my physical limitations. In fact, that had always been the case. I was more determined than most. I don't know why but I have always been like that. That's what made getting sick so hard. All summer long I worked out three or four hours a day, every day. Going into "two a day" nobody was in better shape. All of that hard work went back to zero. So here I am on a Friday, after only 4 days of practice getting ready for the game. Between school and my first week of practice I was extremely tired. On the Friday of the game, one of my teachers who was also one of the football coaches told me to go to the nurse's office to get some sleep. I missed my last few classes that day. I think I sleep for three hours, a fact that I don't think anyone knew. Feeling a little better it was time for the pep rally then travel to the game. The game is about to start and I'm on the sideline. As promised the other guy was starting. About halfway through the first quarter one of the offensive linemen got hurt. Immediately, I got my starting position and they move the other guy to fill the injured player's position.  We were playing well on offense but getting killed on defense. They were either collapsing down on the defensive end and running a sweep or kicking him out and running inside getting 20 or 30 yards every play. From the sideline I could tell what they were doing and keep begging the coach to put me in because I knew I could stop it. It wasn't until the second half and many touchdowns by the other team later, that the coach finally put me in on defense. The first play I got in I knew it was coming right my way. Instead of staying on the line of scrimmage I went straight in the back field and took on the lead blocker. I pushed off of him and tackled the running back for a five-yard loss. It was the first time in the game that we had stopped that play. The second play I'm in, they decide to run the same play and again I stopped them. And again, and again. Finally, they decide to run the same play but the opposite way from me. They had some success but not as much as before. The whole second half I went both ways on offense and defense. We caught up some but unfortunately, we lost the game. After the game the team circles up to get yelled at by the coach. Now I was exhausted. It felt like I had played four games back-to-back. I could barely kneel. I'm in the very back and the coach is yelling and then walks around the circle and comes up to me. He picks me up like a rag doll and says, "if you guys had half the heart of this man, we would have won the game." I'll never forget that. It showed me that with hard work and determination I could achieve. The next three games were the best of my life. The next game I scored two touchdowns and rushed for 134 yards. (I know I play guard. They put in a few plays for me to use my speed)

We beat our school rivals for the first time in 17 years. Probably one of the biggest underdog stories you would ever see. I could probably write a full chapter about that game but that's not what this book is about. I had four incredible games to finish the season. It was bitter sweet because that would be the last time, I played football. Looking back, it was for the best. At the time I was really too small to play in college. After high school I still only weighted 170 lbs. which is way too small to play anything but wide receiver and although I was fast, I wasn't that fast. Plus, I had over ten concussions in high school and playing college could have really screwed me up. There is a song by Garth Brooks that sums it up "Unanswered Prayers". As bad as I wanted to play college football it was a blessing in disguised that I didn't. Now coming to terms with that at the time was very difficult. It was the first time that I had put my mind to something and that it didn't work. All my athletic success in grade school and high school happened when I worked really hard. And through most my life if I set out to do something and worked hard enough, I could make it happen. Instead of looking at it liked I failed I looked at it like a pivot. So, after high school I had to pivot. More about that later. After football, it was time to get ready for track season. Well, I had many months before the season would start but there was off season to get prepared. I think I felt like I still had something to prove since my football season had been cut short. I went to the track coach to write an off-season workout. He wrote one of the hardest workouts you would ever see. I don't think he thought it was a workout someone could or would do. Well, I did it, religiously. When track season started, I was already in tip top shape. Just like in football the first day of practice was kind of easy for me. My track coach couldn't believe it. He asked what I did and I told him I did the workout he gave me. He couldn't believe it. I was all ready for the first track meet. I ran the 200 and 400 meters. But back then we called it the two twenty and the four forty. And as everybody knows the 400 meters is the hardest race. It is a full sprint for a quarter mile. I have always been drawn to the hardest think possible. I don't really know why, I guess it's the challenge of it or that I always had something to prove. From a very early age I always wanted to be the best in whatever I do. I don't know why but that feeling has always been there. My parents weren't like that, so I don't know why I'm like that. It's not a problem unless I'm a bad sport or let it destroy me. I will admit that growing up I did take a loss in sports very hard. Never a bad sport but man I didn't like to lose. Even when my Dallas Cowboys would lose on Sunday, I would have a bad day on Monday. I have since realized that it really is only a game and I don't get too worked up about it anymore. That said, I still try to be the best at personal training, massage and acting.

Now back to the story. It looked like I was going to have a good season in track. I was fast but not the fastest. In the years I ran track from grade school to high school the best I finished was either third or fourth. I had no illusion that I was going to finish first. I usually finished a second or second and a half behind first place. You might not know this unless you know track or watch the Olympics but one second in the 400 meter is about ten yards. Even though I worked my tail off I didn't think I could win state or anything. I guess I just wanted to be the best I could be. Unlike other sports I didn't get that upset about losing. Mainly, because when you sprint a quarter mile and you give it everything you have and you feel like you are going to die you don't care too much about where you finished, you're just glad that you didn't die.

The season started and I was doing better than I had ever done. To be honest I don't remember all of that season. It was 30 years ago. But I do remember half way through that season I pulled my hamstring. Kind of an important muscle when it comes to running. I missed a few track meets but started getting ready for the state meet. I still didn't know how I would do but I wanted to do my best. I wasn't the best but I tried to outwork everybody else. Kind of always been my mantra. Something I still do till this day. I remember it was a cool day in Dallas when we had a practice that was a week before the state meet. It was perfect training weather, not too cold but not hot so I could run without getting overheated. It was toward the end of practice and I was finishing up on the 200 meters. We would run one at full speed then rest and do it again and again. I don't remember how many times I ran the 200 meters but I do remember running really good times. The coached said last one. I really wanted it to be my fastest one yet. I took off well out of the blocks. I was flying and then it happened. The event that would change my life forever. Through the second turn, when I reached top speed, my hamstring snapped. It tore from the bottom close to the knee and from the top of the hamstring that attaches to the hip under the butt. The hamstring collapsed in the middle of the upper leg. It's called "cantalouping." Either that or I just made up that word but it describes it perfectly. The hamstring balls up in the middle of the upper leg in the shape of a cantaloupe. When someone is moving at top speed it's very hard to know what is happening. The body is an amazing machine. When the hamstring snapped there was no decision, I didn't think "oh I better slow down I think something happened." My body simply would not let me put my foot back down which is a big problem when traveling at a high rate of speed. I just went down, face first and slid around five lines of the track and ended up in the grass. Now you have to realize all of it was involuntary. None of it was my idea. The best way I can describe it is like a car blowing a tire. It just happens and seconds later you are in the ditch. So, there I am in the ditch and I can't move. I know something major has happened but I'm kind of out of it. It's like I almost passed out but I was awake. Later I would realize I was in shock. There was pain but not tons, at first. That's what is good about shock it keeps you from feeling all the pain. But you can also die from shock if the injury is very traumatic. I don't remember much of what came after, but I do remember that it took four people to carry me to the field house. How I got home and the rest of the night is fussy but I do remember lots and lots of pain.

I couldn't walk at all. The next day I wrapped it with an ace bandage and grab some crutches (I think we had some) and went to school. Yeah, that's right I went to school the next day after a major injury. Back then we didn't go to the hospital or doctor unless something was hanging off, like when I cut my finger in the lawn mower. I think at some point I went to the doctor or the physical therapist or both. Looking back, I definitely needed to have surgery to re-attach the hamstring but there again back then you would only have surgery if you were dying. Within a week I was doing rehab. I went to the physical therapist every day for months. For those who don't know when you tear a muscle the area around the muscle turns black and blue and other fun colors. Since the hamstring is the back of the upper leg and I couldn't always keep my leg elevated the black and blue runs down the leg and into the foot. It's just a horrible sight. It eventually goes away but I think it was six to eight weeks. I don't remember in detail the rehab but I do remember it was long, painful and interesting. As I have stated I have had tons of injuries but this was the worse so far and still remains one of the top injuries I have ever had. Through the rehab process I started to learn more about the body and became interested in physical fitness. With-in a few months I could jog and workout but till this day I have problems with that hamstring. Years after the injury the physical therapist tested the hamstring and said that I had about half a hamstring. Surprisingly I could still run, play basketball, and even sprint. I just have to be careful not to overdue and to really warm it up before taxing it. So that was the end of my sports career in high school. Not a success story. No "overcoming the odds story", that led to a professional football career. Not out with a bang but a whimper. Like most stories of a kid wanting a professional sports career it wasn't to be. It was a blessing in disguise even if I didn't know it at the time. But all of it, the injuries, the pain, the mono, the disappointment would all serve me for what was to come next.

As my senior year was winding down the only thing left to do was organize prom. You see I was senior class president and I was in charge of prom. Like so many things in my life I had no idea what I was doing. But I was going to just "fake it until you make it". If I have ever wanted to do something, learn something, change something, I would just figure it out. Ask people, read about it, or whatever it took to get the job done. Now if you want to know how to do something there is a YouTube video for it. But back then before the internet (yes there was a time where there was no information highway) we had to do things the hard way. I did have help. We had teachers that I could ask and we had student counsel but the heavy lifting was up to me. Getting the location, getting the music, raising the money, decorations, and everything else. It was a lot of work. So much so that I forgot to get a date to the prom. At that time, I didn't have a girlfriend so there was no automatic date. Two weeks before prom I asked a friend that I had known from grade school and she said yes and we had a really good time. Not to brag but one of our teachers said it was the best prom they had seen. I was very proud of my accomplishment because I had worked so hard on it and it was a huge success. I think people in my class took notice of it and voted me prom king. I know, I know how it sounds but it wasn't because I was "popular" it's because I worked hard and followed through with what I committed to do. I was never an asshole. I talked to everybody and treated my classmates with respect. I wasn't the asshole high school jock that is portrayed in every movie and TV show. I'm sure there were people that didn't like me and there were people I didn't care for but that is true in life. The funny thing is I have no idea why I wanted to be class president. I have always reached for what seems to be impossible odds. If it is tough to do, I'm in. I have always wanted to defy the odds. I ran the 400 meters because it was the hardest race, I started my own business at 22 years old because that was a hard thing to do. And then pursuing acting is probably the hardest thing to do.  I have always had the idea to do something and then figure out how to do it later. Kind of like writing this book. Even though I don't know why I wanted to be class president it has benefited me for the rest of my life. The skills I learned on how to put something together, how to organize something, and have it turn out to be very successful was a boost in confidence. If I set my mind to something, I can achieve it. Now obviously it didn't happen when it came to a football career but there are other factors at play there.

# Chapter Three

## The College Years

The end of high school was bittersweet. Most people were going off to a big college and I knew I would be staying home and going to a community college. My parents at the time couldn't afford to send me to college. I kind of knew this the whole time I was in high school. Maybe that's the reason I tried so hard in sports. I knew that my grades weren't going to get me a scholarship, so maybe I could get a football scholarship. Towards the end of senior year, I knew that I would be staying home and going to a community college and have to work. At the time, I had no clue what I was going to do. In high school I seemed to be the go-to guy if you had problems. Wise beyond my years I was told and continue to be told that until this day. I could always help others with their problem but not my own and that continues to be the case now. I thought I would be a therapist. One of the classes I enrolled in was psychology. So maybe this would be what I would do. And I signed up for a few more classes and then came my elective. Ballet. Wait what. There was something else that was burning inside of me. In 1987 there was a little movie called "Dirty Dancing". As you know I was in all four musicals in high school and was interested in acting. Patrick

Swayze was amazing. He played football growing up and did ballet. He was a dancer but a man's man. That's what I wanted to do. Plus, he got all the women and that's what I wanted too. Because of Patrick Swayze, I signed up for my first ballet class. At the same time, I went to a dance studio to do partner dancing. They were so surprised that an 18-year-old male wanted to dance that they gave me lessons for free. I got a partner and we competed in ballroom. And yes, we did the "dirty dancing" dance from the movie for competition. The lift overhead and everything. We even practice the lift in water just like in the movie. At the same time, I got a local "talent agent" in Dallas. I put that in quotes because I'm not sure how legit they were. Mainly, I would do extra work here and there. I don't remember this, but my mother told me when I was little that I said I wanted to be two things when I grew up. Roger Staubach (quarterback for the Dallas Cowboys) or Dick Van Dike. I grew up loving "The Carol Burnett Show". So much so that one time at my grandparents' house I put on "The John Show".  I'm sure it was terrible but after the show I passed a hat around so they could put money in it, because I wanted to be paid for my work after all. Since the Roger Staubach thing didn't pan out, I guess I would try to be Dick Van Dike. With all that going on I still needed to find work but what would that be? Right after high school a few of my friends and I worked for Texas Auto Prep. They put in air conditioners, car alarms, car phones, pretty much everything that comes standard in a car now-a-days. In 1988 all of that was after market stuff. Our job was to drive the beat-up old cars to the dealerships leave the keys in the floor board and pick up the car that needed whatever. We were picking up brand new cars and high-end cars. It was a blast. It was only hard because of the Texas summer heat. I remember we got paid four bucks an hour, which was more than any job I had before. Through high school I made minimum wage, $3.35 an hour. Four bucks, wow! That was a good summer job between high school and college. I got to hang out with my friends before they went off to college. But I needed to find something else when school started in the fall. One day that summer I ran into a friend of mine's brother. I knew him but not well. He was telling me that he was a floor trainer at a gym. They had a fire and were reopening and needed some trainers. That sounded really cool to me. I went down and applied and got the job. I didn't start right away because it wouldn't open for another month which was about the same time, I started college. And this is where my story really begins.

When I went into Rock White Athletic Club for the first time it was under construction. Remodeling after a fire and a change in ownership. There were two new owners, Bob and Dee. They were from the real estate field and wanted to try their hand in the fitness field. This was 1988 and the fitness field was starting to boom. Step aerobics, high impact aerobics, and personal training were just becoming main stream. Personal training was around in the early 80's just not a profession, yet. Personal trainers were mainly in the body building world. Aerobics was already main stream but personal training was yet to be main stream. What was big was nautilus. About 15 machines in a circuit. Downstairs there were the locker rooms, four racquetball courts, a huge aerobics room, a nursery, an indoor/outdoor pool, offices, and a snack bar. Upstairs was the fitness floor with the nautilus circuit, free weights, cardio machines, and a raised track that was 10 laps per mile. With my limited life experience this place was amazing. It also had a steam room, wool pool, and dry sauna. It was the coolest place I had ever seen. I was friendly and out-going and was afraid of nothing when I was 18. I had been working since the six grade. I had been on many interviews for jobs in high school, so I was prepared when it came time to interview for a "real job". I can't stress enough how important it was to have a job as a kid. It taught me a lot that prepared me for the real world. I kind of had to work because we didn't have lots of money growing up. But I think it was a blessing in disguise. I think all high school kids should have a job. There are things you learn that you can't in school, "real world experience". That is something you can't learn in books. How to interview, how to deal with others, how to "sale" yourself, the value of a dollar, and so much more.  I truly believe that having a job in high school gave me the confidence to land the job as a "floor trainer". I had no experience. I had no business getting that job but I didn't know that I shouldn't get that job. I was confident and had a go-getter attitude. I was willing to learn and practically talked my way into that job. When I started, I remember making $4.75 an hour. That's more than I had ever made. At the time minimum wage was still $3.25 so I thought I hit the jackpot. I remember starting out I was an eager beaver. I was going to soak up everything I could. I knew how to work out. I was an athlete in high school, I was a power lifter in high school so I knew a little. But never knew how to teach someone to workout. The fitness director took us through two days of training. Not super extensive just mainly how to take someone through the nautilus machines. We had these cards to write down the machines and what weights to use and how many reps and sets to do. Very basic stuff. I remember the first few days after we opened were very boring. A lot of cleaning. Getting ready for people to sign up. It didn't take long for things to pick up. People that use to be a member started to come back. There was a big marketing campaign to get new members and they started to pour in by the carload. Quickly I would be giving tours because the sales director was so busy that they needed other employees to take people on a tour of the gym. I was really good at that because I loved the gym so much, it wasn't even like I was selling. I was just showing a friend the coolest place on earth. I think I had a 100% success rate. I probably didn't but it felt like I did. They were very few people that didn't sign up right then and there. I didn't hard sell anyone. If they wanted to think about it, I said that was great, no problem. Most the time they came back. The best part was I made a commission on every sale. I don't remember how much but it helped. I worked about 35 hours a week. I had the 4pm-10pm shift and Saturday 8am-2pm. I was making around $800 dollars a month give or take. Enough to live on barely.  At the time I was living at home and paying for college which wasn't much since I was going to a community college. The fall semester of 1988 I took an algebra class and the before mentioned, psychology class, and ballet. I was failing algebra so I had to drop it. Ballet was great because I was one of two guys and the only straight guy. All the girls were so amazed that a straight guy was taking ballet I got a lot of attention from the beautiful girls. As I said before I also was doing some extra work. Extra work is basically background people you see in movies and TV shows. There wasn't a lot of shows that were shooting in Dallas except for the show "Dallas". It was toward the end of the run of the show. But this was my first acting job. I had to go downtown next to the Palms restaurant and walk from one street corner to the next. And then do that over and over again. Then came my big break. Me and the woman they paired me with, were grabbed and told to go inside the restaurant. They needed two people to walk through the restaurant with the camera on us and then the camera would stop on Sue Ellen and Patrick Duffy, the first two celebrities I would ever see. I was nervous but all we had to do is walk 10 feet. They said action and we walked. Three steps in, they yelled cut because our dress shoes were making too much noise on the wood floor. What most people don't know is movie sets are very quiet. Even in a restaurant scene. The background actors or "extras" are supposed to move their mouths but not speak. You are to use your fork and knife but not make a sound. That's so you can hear the main actors talk. All the background sounds and voices are put in later called looping. Which is exactly like it sounds, they loop in the sounds later.

Our walk had to be quiet. The second take, they told us just walk on your tip toes. On action we started walking on our tip toes and then cut, cut. The camera guy yells it looks like they are walking on their tip toes. At the time I thought I was screwing up and was for sure going to get fired right then and there. My acting career would be over before it started. What I realized later is, it had nothing to do with us. They are just trying to figure out how to get the shot. They decided to have us take our shoes off and walk normal. Success. We did it and they went on with the scene. We did it maybe another five times. And then we were done. This was my first time I could be seen on T.V., all of three seconds of it. Yep, all that for three seconds. But I was in show biz. I made $35 dollars for the day which I think was about ten hours. The rest of that fall I would go to school and work at the athletic club and dance at the studio. Then in January I got an extra job that would change my life.

It was 1989 the year that "Born on the Fourth of July" was being filmed and for some reason they were filming in Dallas. I got the call from my "agent" and I jumped at the chance to be in a "Hollywood film". Now for those of you who don't know it can get quite cold in Dallas Texas in the winter. Usually, at least one ice storm or snow storm and cold every season. The extra job was for a student at a college, protesting the Vietnam War, outside! It was cold that day. I think in the 30's but the wind was blowing so the wind chill was in the teens. The catch is, the scene takes place in the spring so no coats or hats, just a long sleeve shirt and pants. I was smart enough to put thermals under my clothes which helped but 14 hours outside in that weather was still cold. Tom Cruise was the biggest star at the time. He was coming off of making Top Gun and Rain Man and this was going to be his Oscar role, which he did get a nomination. It was exciting. I never saw a huge movie star before. As extras we were told before Tom Cruise came out of his trailer that we were not to talk to him and not to even look at him in the eyes. Well, that seemed a little snobby at the time. It has been reported over the years that certain celebrities ask not to be looked at in the eyes. It seems very stuck up until you realize the reason.  I have learned over the years the amazing amount of concentration it takes to really pull off a difficult acting scene. To pull off an emotional scene or a scene where you have to be angry takes a lot of concentration. Talking to someone or ever looking at someone can throw you off. The last thing you need is an extra coming up to you and distracting you. I think it's individual. Some people can laugh and joke right up to action and then just cry their eyes out. But most can't do that. I will say that not every scene needs super concentration. They are times that I can be friendly and outgoing before a scene and sometimes I need to concentrate.  I politely tell the person that I need to concentrate and most the time they understand. Now if a celebrity says they don't want people to talk to them or look them in the eyes in day-to-day life then maybe they are just an asshole. Now, back to the story.

They make the announcement about Tom and a few minutes later he appears. He comes out of his trailer in character with his head down and a very serious look on his face. The first thing I noticed is how short he was. You always think they are going to be bigger. You see them on the big screen and they look huge. But trust me they are all smaller than you think. Even the "big guy" in the movie is smaller than you think. I stood next to Jean Claude van Damme on the movie "Universal Soldier: The Return" for over ten hours. He is all of 5'5 maybe 140 lbs. You probably think I'm lying. He is extremely lean and very muscular, so on camera he looks big. In the scene he had to walk down these stairs and then walk up to another actor. Right before he gets to the other actor he has to step up on an apple box so he can be eye to eye with the actor. It's movie magic.

After Tom Cruise went by, I only saw him at a distance the rest of the day. Mostly I remember the cold and how poorly extras are treated on set. Come to find out extras are the lowest thing on set. The furniture is more important and they make you feel that way. They even have different food for the extras than the rest of the cast and crew. It's not bad just a lot less quality than the other food. It's a chance for a human to know what it's like to be cattle. Extras also eat last. Now that sounds mean but there is an actual purpose for that. The cast and crew have to eat then get ready for the next scene.

Maybe it's wardrobe change or setting up lights. But they have to be ready when lunch is over so it makes since that they eat first. But how extras can be treated or talked to is very degrading. Almost like they aren't human. But because of that it can be a bonding experience for the extras. Remember this is 1989, no cell phones and no internet so people had to actually talk to each other to past the time. Or you could read a book but that was hard to do on this set. Halfway through the day I was getting what they call "punch drunk". I was very out going back then and talkative but being "punch drunk" I was in rare form. I was making a group of people laugh and laugh. The more they laughed the more it encouraged me. We talked and laughed for hours and hours. I remember they finally let us hang out inside. There was no heat but at least it saved us from the wind. We all huddled together to keep warm. It's amazing how close people can get in a short period of time. When the day was finally over, we didn't want the friendship to end. We all exchanged numbers to stay in touch. The one thing I left out is that the group of people were all in a two-year musical theatre program at Mountain View college. This encounter would change my life. I know people say that but this really did send me on the path towards acting. I would stay in touch with them but mainly with one of them. His name was Dewey. We got along great and became friends. At the time I was living with two roommates, friends from high school. This is before the age of cell phones so we had a land line with an answering machine. Hard to believe but you would only get your messages when you were home. I didn't think much about it but Dewey was quite flamboyant and he would leave quit flamboyant messages on the answering machine which my roommates would hear. So obviously they assumed I was gay even though I had a beautiful girlfriend. I was very naive when I was young and really didn't know what "gay" was. It bothered me that they thought I was gay, not because I had a problem with it but because they made me feel like it was a negative. At the time I barely understood what gay was. I knew it was when someone liked someone of the same sex. I don't remember having a feeling about it one way or another. But I didn't want to be called gay because I wasn't and people made it a negative thing. All I knew is I liked Dewey he was funny and we got along well and I started not to care what others thought. I knew who I was and who I liked. I was very curious about what gay was. I wasn't really exposed to gay people when I was growing up. Or I didn't think I was. Looking back, I had relatives that are gay, my theater teacher was gay and other students were gay but I didn't know. Back in the 70's and 80's most people were in the closet and openly gay people were not on  T.V. It was there just not talked about. I listened to Queen and Boy George and was none the wiser.

Like I said, naive.  There was never an open dialog about people who were gay. Times have really changed for the better although we have a long way to go.

Bringing up Dewey is an important point to the story because I had a choice to be friends with him or to feel pressure from my roommates and not be friends. I know I made the right decision for so many reasons. A few months into our friendship he asked me if I wanted to audition for the musical theatre program. It was a small program which only took 15 students and was only for two years. It was invitation only to audition so I felt honored. It would be a huge commitment.

The classes went from 8am-3:30pm Monday-Friday. I worked 4pm to 10pm Monday-Friday so it was a huge decision, but first I had to audition which I haven't done but a few times before.

Singing has never been my thing. I never had a lesson except for the musicals in high school. But those weren't really lessons just trying to get high school kids to learn a song and not suck. To audition for the musical theater program at Mountain View College I would have to sing and read a monologue. Still to this day it was the worse audition I have ever done. And I have had some real stinkers over the years. It was so bad that they just had me sing happy birthday. Not only was it bad but embarrassing. I left there thinking well that was a waste of time. On the day I meet Dewey several of the others that I met were also in the program with Dewey. They must have all put in a good word for me because somehow, I was accepted. In the fall of 1989, I would embark on a path that would lead me to where I am today.

## Chapter Four

## A New Beginning

I was nervous to embark on this new journey. I knew I really wanted to be an actor but I haven't really done it. I did four musicals in high school, mainly ensemble, which really means I danced in the background and said one or two lines. I wasn't a good enough singer so I couldn't get one of the main parts. And the only other experience I had was the few extra jobs I got after high school. This was going to be a tough thing going to school from 8:00 am - 3:30 and then work 4:00-10:00pm. And also work 8:00am-2:00pm on Saturday. Thank God I was young and had lots of energy because I wouldn't be able to do that schedule later in life.  But at this time, I really wasn't having any real back issues. I had pain in my back just like in high school but it didn't really prohibit me. Oddly, at this time I kind of thought that back pain was normal. I thought that everybody had it. I asked my best friend one time if everything hurts when he wakes up in the morning and he said ,no he feels great. Oddly, that was the first time I realized what I was experiencing was different than others.

Since it's been almost 30 years, I don't remember in detail my first day of the performing arts musical theatre program or PAMTP. I do remember they stressed how important it was to be there day one. And when we found out that two out of the sixteen classmates were going to be two days late, everybody was pissed. Now the two being late were performing at a summer stock theatre and was driving across country to get here. I remember day three the best. Halfway through our first class the two students show up. Beth and Scott. Beth said hello and sat down and Scott preceded to go around the class and personally introduce himself to everybody by shaking hands vigorously while staring through your soul. I thought he was going to break my hand and burn a whole in the back of my head. I remember thinking who is this jagweed. He's one of the fakest people I've ever met. As it turns out I was wrong. I just have never met a more upbeat and positive person. Also, I later found out that they had been driving day and night to get here and was hopped up on tons of caffeine which made him bigger than life. The reason this is in the story is that he quickly became my best friend and continues to be 30 years later. Most the time my first impressions of someone is correct but this time I was wrong. But Scott has heard this before. He is bigger than life. It's just who he is. Thankfully, over the years he has brought it down some but still one of the happiest and positive people you will ever met.  We quickly get in a rhythm of school. It was strange to be in college and have to be there from 8am-3:30pm. It was a lot like high school from that respect. The program was unique in the fact that all 16 students took every class together. We didn't see or have anything to do with other students at the college. The theatre department was kind of separate from the rest of the school. It was a very different situation. It's amazing how close people can get when you spend that much time with each other. Not only the school hours but after school rehearsals and going out on the weekends. It was very much like high school in the fact that we had this shared experience. Most of us are still in contact (at least on Facebook) until this day.

My life back then was very complicated.  I was going to school full time, working full time, and in a serious relationship. It was quit overwhelming to say the lease. I did really love my girlfriend but I was only 20 years old and had no idea about my future. Was I going to move to New York or Los Angeles to go for the acting? Was I going to stay in Dallas and be a fitness guy?  With all of this I was still just a 20-year-old kid trying to figure it out. With all the good qualities I had I was still immature. I really couldn't handle everything. As good of a loving relationship I was in, I wasn't ready and screwed it all up. She once said to me, "I wish we met later in life." Oh, how right she was. Still until this day she is one of the great loves of my life. Due to how painful this situation was for me; in the famous words of Forrest Gump, "That's all I got to say about that."

The first semester was the hardest. I was not musically inclined or very good at dance or for that matter I couldn't act my way out of a paper bag. But I wanted to be good. I tried very hard. I was OK at dancing, mainly because I was fit and limber and had some training. I loved acting but just hadn't had too many experiences doing it. And singing. Oh, how I wanted to be good but the fear of singing so overwhelmed me my throat would close up and I would end up sounding like Kermit the frog, but not in a good way. Over the years I have accepted that singing isn't going to be my thing. I can sort of carry a tune now but I won't be headlining a musical on Broadway anytime soon. I have strength and rhythm and could dance some but not well enough to be a dancer on Broadway. So that left acting. I have done quite a bit of theatre and have been good at it. But as a naturally shy person (most close friends wouldn't say I'm shy) and a quiet talker, it took a lot of effort to perform on stage. That's when I found acting on camera. It felt the best of all the arts program. The emotion is all in the face, you don't have to be loud so the whole theatre can hear you, and you connect to the person or persons that I'm in the scene with instead of cheating out to the audience. This felt the best to me.

When the first semester was over, we got a one-on-one evaluation from the teachers. You sit in a chair in the middle of the stage with the panel of teachers in front of you. I don't remember most of it but the one thing I do remember is the head of the program, Rod, stood up and throw his hands in the air and said, "I have no idea what to do with you!" and walked out. Which translated to "You are the worst thing we have ever seen." In fairness, he was probably right. But I was trying my best and really, really wanted to be good, so this was devastating. I was so upset that the other teachers could tell and were trying to soften the blow. I really did think of quitting but I've never quit on anything I have ever started. I might have changed directions but never quit. Over the Christmas break I had a lot of thinking to do. I didn't think about quitting for very long. I was determined that I would show him. How dare he say that. I worked and worked that whole semester. At the end of the first year, we had to put together a one man show with acting, singing, and dancing, that we wrote, directed, and produced. Of course, we got help from our teachers but we had to put it all together and perform it in front of an audience.

It's the day of the shows. We each did our own show I think they were 5 minutes each, and we could have two or three other students in our show. So not only were we doing our own show we would be in others as well. Everything was going smoothly and then it was time for my show. I was nervous but also clam in a strange way. I felt prepared and ready. The show starts with me singing happy birthday to myself because I was alone. My show was mainly about being alone and wanting to be with someone. Oddly, is what I'm still going through today. More about that later. And yes, if you were paying attention that was the song I sang to get into the program.  The irony is not lost on me. I sing happy birthday and do my little woe is me speech and then comes the big song and dance break. I can't remember the song I sang or any of the dance moves but I do remember what happened next. About 15 seconds into the song all, and I mean all, the lights go out. Pitch black. Can't see one foot in front of me. But it was drilled into our heads no matter what, under any circumstances; come on everybody say it with me, "THE SHOW MUST GO ON" so I kept singing and dancing around the room, can't see a damn thing, and David Rogers continues playing the piano like nothing happened. He is so good; he could play the piano blindfolded in a hail storm.  Now, unknown to the crowd, I had two girls come on stage and dance with me. Since they didn't sing the crowd didn't know they were on stage. We do the whole number in the dark and finish. No one claps. All you hear is Rod. He stands up and yells, "What the fuck happened to the lights!" And the guy in the booth said that the whole panel went down and he couldn't do anything. "Then turn on the house lights for fucks sake", Rod yells. Now mind you we have just finished a dance number that took us all over the stage and two girls are next to me when we finished doing jazz hands or something like it. When the house lights come on the audience see's three people on stage doing jazz hands sweating and breathing hard, so it's no wonder that they started laughing. I didn't take it personally at all. I know it was ridiculous looking and I did nothing wrong. It sucked but I didn't feel that bad. I know it's not my fault. They said they would have to take a break to fix the problem. I was cool with that. I told someone that I would go in the back and collect my thoughts and to come and get me when they were ready. Well, apparently no one said anything so when they were ready for me, nobody could find me. Someone had said I had run off. Apparently, they looked for me for a while before they found me so when I returned to the stage, I got a big ovation which was a little embarrassing. I started again and started to sing happy birthday but I stopped and said, "you guys know how it goes" and moved on with the show which got me a good laugh. The rest of my show went well. I was told later that the whole panel going out has never happened before and it didn't happen for anyone else's show. I don't know if that was an omen to get out of the business or a sign to overcome obstacles but that dichotomy still puzzles me today.  I did get a good grade and Rod said I had made the most improvement out of anyone in the program. So maybe I could do this. But things are about to get a lot harder.

Although I had a full-time job and was going to school full time, I was still just a kid. I was mature in a lot of ways but still at 20 years old I wanted to have fun and party. I was good at partying. I threw great parties and was the life of the party. I'm shy by nature but with a little liquid courage I was a social butterfly. I was living on my own by the age of 19 and had bills and responsibilities that other kids my age didn't. Most of my friends were off to college and didn't have to work and did what most kids in college do, party. I was not immune to being a kid even though I was growing up fast. The long and short of it is I partied too hard on a Friday night, oversleep and was late in opening the gym and got fired. I had worked my ass off at this gym and one mistake I was gone. Deservingly so I will admit now but then I thought I was being wronged. On top of that my relationship was ending and I needed to find a new place to live and a new job. Now the relationship that was ending was devastating and extremely painful. I take full responsibility for my part but I was too immature to handle it correctly. I found a job waiting tables at a restaurant called By George.  It was a cool hip restaurant on Greenville Avenue. A street that had lots of great restaurants and bars for miles. The restaurant was in the heart of Greenville Avenue. I started a few weeks before school started back up. I had just moved out of my girlfriends and into my own apartment. My first apartment by myself. I really needed to feel like I could take care of myself. I had gone from my parents to my sisters to living with two roommates to living with my girlfriend. I needed to stand on my own two feet even though I still loved my girlfriend I just needed time to figure me out. To this day I don't regret that decision, just how I handled it. I think I was to mature for my own good in some ways. I was in a grown-up relationship at 19 but still had no idea who I was. Losing my job was not part of the plan, I just had to make the most of it. So new job, new place, and new semester what could go wrong.

School was going OK. I picked up where I left off. I was in a groove so everything was going OK there. But waiting tables was not the dream job of an actor that I'd hope it would be. I was use to going straight from school to work with no time off, ever. Now I'm waiting tables three or four times a week including weekends so I have more free time on my hands than I've ever had and had less money than ever before. I thought I could make more money waiting tables with less time but I was mistaken.  Normally you could make good money waiting tables but not me. I was really living Murphy's Law. Everything went wrong. It seemed like every shift something bad would happen. I would have a big party of ten come in and take up most of my section and stay most of the night and leave me a dollar for a tip. Now at the time in 1990 in Texas waiters made $2.01 an hour, just barely enough to cover taxes. Most of the money you made was in tips. A dollar a night wouldn't cut it. Now most nights weren't that bad but it seemed like I was cursed. One time after waiting awhile for my drinks to come out (because they ordered six long island iced teas, which are difficult to make) I rounded the corner and another waiter ran into me spilling all of my drinks which means we had to start all over again. When I finally got the drinks out to her, she gave me the dirtiest look and said "it took you long enough" and then stiffed me.  And that stuff would happen to me all the time. In hindsight I should have realized that this was the universe telling me to get out of there but I wasn't as "in tuned" back then as I am now. I waited tables the whole fall semester but I knew something had to change. For some reason I keep thinking that I needed to get my job back at the gym. That thought would set me up for the rest of my life. It was December and the semester was ending. I was so broke that I knew that I couldn't continue that way for another semester. I had an idea to meet the owner that didn't fire me for a beer. He agreed and I somehow talked him into giving me another shot. It might have been the alcohol but I'll take it. The only problem was I couldn't afford school so with one semester left in the program I had to drop out. I regret that until this day but it had to be done. Getting my job back was pivotal to how my story goes. At the time I still didn't know how important that would become. Without that happening I wouldn't have become a personal trainer and I wouldn't have had the means to pursue an acting career.

I started back at my job where I left off but with a little more maturity. I found out when I came back that there had been a backlash of me being fired and the members were complaining. I worked harder than most and was very liked by the members. I think I was hired back so people would stop with the complaints. It's amazing if you work hard and are kind to people, they will go to the mat for you. It was the first time that I felt that kind of support but it wouldn't be the last. Now things seem to be getting back on track but I was still grieving the end of a significant relationship. I started boxing and working out like a monster. Since I didn't have school, I would work out for three hours a day. Yep, really. An hour and a half of weights, 30 minutes of abs, and an hour of cardio. I'm exhausted just writing that now. But I got in the best shape of my life. And then biometrics started. Biometrics was a program that was starting at the gym. It was known as the super slow protocol. A 30-minute weight training program with the nautilus equipment with a diet plan. They needed trainers to take people through the program so I signed up. I believe the pay was $10 for each 30-minute session which was

$20 an hour. Three times what I would normally make. It didn't take me long to realize that this personal training field was the way to go. At the time I realized that if I wanted to pursue acting, I needed to have a job that was flexible and paid the most it could per hour so I wouldn't have to work 10-hour days to live. Something that I still believe 30 years later.

After the biometrics program was over most people wanted to continue with a trainer. Now this is 1991 and personal training wasn't really a profession. The words personal trainer was out there and it was only for body builders and athletes. This was the days when high impact aerobics and leg warmers was the thing. In fact, there was no certification for personal trainers, only for aerobics instructors.  All the clients I took through the program wanted to continue and that's the moment that personal training began. There wasn't a book or any reference on how to do it. It seemed like all around the country that personal training started to take hold. But it was such a new field for the main stream market. Of course, personal training had been around since the 1970's but it exploded in the 90's. I can't quit remember how many people I first started with but it wasn't more than five clients. Some wanted to continue with exactly what they were doing, a 30-minute super slow protocol, which I did. But quickly I got my clients to see the benefit of changing it up and got them to do an hour of training. I believe that I charged $25 an hour which was a ton of money at the time. I still worked 40 hours for the club and trained my clients when I was off. I worked very hard and practically lived at the gym.  Just as the personal training started my mentor, the fitness director, was leaving. He was going to med school. I hadn't been working back at the gym for very long but I felt that I would be the best person to take over the fitness director's job. I was still only 20 years old but I had tons of energy and a lot of unearned confidence and thought nothing of putting my hat in the ring. I remember putting together a big proposal. Rallied the members to get behind me, and wouldn't take no for an answer. Now the owners didn't want me and they made that very clear. But I was a pain in the ass. The position required a degree and would never go to someone as young as me, I was 20 years old almost 21. I'm not sure exactly how I got the job but I did, making me the youngest fitness director in Dallas and maybe anywhere. I became a salary employee and I remember it came out to $8.25 an hour which was double what I was making.  Now it was time to enact my plan, start a personal training program.

## Chapter Five

## Personal Training

I've just turned 21 and became the fitness director of a 3,000-membership club. I had already been doing personal training but wanted to advertise and create a program and add trainers.  The year is 1991 and there isn't a certification for personal training. The organization I.D.E.A. (international dance and exercise association) had a certification for aerobics instructors. I heard that they were going to offer a personal training certification and I signed up immediately. If you studied the materials and then took the test and passed, anybody could say they are a certified trainer. Let's just say the bar was low. I wanted to be good at what I do and I have a passion for fitness, so I continued to read, talk to other trainers, and just try to absorb as much info as I could.  Within the year a new certification was available through A.C.E. (American Council of Exercise). And for some reason the I.D.E.A. certification was no longer valid. I took the first available test for A.C.E. and was one of 500 trainers across the U.S. to be certified. It's funny to think back and realize I was there at the start of an industry. Personal training wasn't a job before the 90's. Yes, there were trainers in the 80's and even the 70's but not in the main stream. I think the dot.com boom of the 90's gave people more dispensable income. Not to mention fitness became big and the 80's and continued into the 90's. In the early 90's aerobics was king, especially step aerobics. At White Rock Athletic Club, we had the aerobics room on the bottom floor with four racquetball courts and the cardio machines, free weights and nautilus equipment was upstairs. Mainly, it was woman on the first floor and men on the second floor. Now some woman lifted weights and some came upstairs to do cardio and some machines but very few women did weight training. To start a personal training business, I needed to talk a few women into doing weights. A lot of guys didn't do personal training because "they know how to lift weights it's in their DNA". or at least that's what they thought. I would get some male clients but in the beginning my male clients wanted weight loss and general fitness. My big idea was to get women from downstairs to upstairs. Like I said some woman would come upstairs to do the treadmill or the bike so I knew most the members. I was a floor trainer but also the sales guy the toilet cleaner and the whatever else needs to be done guy. I did feel like a host or greeter most the time. I became friends with some of the "aerobics woman" and there was a huge interest in weight lifting but most would tell me they were intimidated by the weight room. I knew if I could get a few women that would let me work with them and talk me up, I could get business. I asked two women that I knew, and offered free personal training. All I asked is that they said good things to members. They were however very fit from years of aerobics and I knew with lifting weights they could easily get some definition. (I wasn't stupid) And that's exactly what happened. Quickly they were getting compliments from other women asking them what they had been doing and of course they laid it on thick. Giving me all the credit, which was nice but I really didn't do that much. But that was my strategy. I didn't have money to advertise so I trained two clients for free and let them do all my advertising and it really worked. One by one women would come upstairs and I became very busy, really quickly. I was still working 40 hours as the fitness director and 20 hours personal training. I couldn't take on more clients so I started to get more trainers. The biggest problem I had was convincing clients to train with another trainer. They heard that I was "the guy" and that's who they wanted. Nice to be popular but it made it hard to grow a business.  At the time, personal training programs were new, and fitness club owners didn't really know the money maker they would become.  I set it up as an 80/20 split. 80% to the trainer and 20% to the club. I'm not exactly sure what we charged but $27 an hour is a number I remember or something close to that. I quickly had five trainers working under me and I had a waiting list of people wanting to train with me.  It was like an overnight boom looking back on it. I know that it wasn't that easy but once we had people sign up the word got out and it was a steady flow of clients. I do remember hitting the 100 hours of personal training a week between the five trainers after just a few months.  At this point, I was just living at the gym. Twelve- or thirteen-hour days. I didn't mind the hours because I loved what I was doing. As the fitness director I had to make sure everything was running smoothly, take care of members, equipment, doing sales, cleaning, staffing, running the personal training program and on top of that I was doing 20 hours of personal training a week. I think my main job was dealing with the owners of the club. In the two and a half years working there I knew more about gyms than they would ever know. They seemed to regret the fact that I was very popular with the members and the members would always back me against management. They were definitely threatened but knew that I was good for business. I don't know when the owners started to have financial troubles but they were starting to make cuts and the writing was on the wall. Knowing that I was valuable to the membership they didn't want to fire me, again, so they combined the general manager position with the fitness director and it made me something like head trainer. This was a big blow because I gave everything to this club almost my life. No really, I really almost died.

It was a Saturday at closing. As I've said before, I had to do just about everything at that club. There was opening the club and closing the club, which had certain things that had to get done. Shocking the pool was something at closing. Putting chlorine in the pool was called shocking the pool. You would go into the maintenance closet, go to this barrel and get two scoops of chlorine and pour it into the pool. Very routine thing I've done many times.  It got a little harder when you were almost out. The chlorine would be hardened at the bottom of the barrel so you would have to chip at it to break it up. We were instructed to use the whole barrel before opening a new one. So, on this day I chipped away to get all the chlorine I could. (Anybody about to guess what's going to happen). The barrel is so tall that half my body is in it. And I just keep chipping away at this hardened mess kicking up a lot of dust. I finally get enough chlorine to "shock the pool" and then I started coughing because of all the dust.  I go into the locker room to get some water and then I couldn't breathe.  What had happened is the second I drank the water it mixed with the chlorine dust and closed my throat.  There are not many people there except for a few employees. I walked toward the front but I couldn't speak. I had my hands around my throat as a sign that I couldn't breathe. We had an oxygen tank around the corner that I keep pointing at but no one could tell what I was pointing at. They laid me down and the last thing I heard was Michelle (the aerobics instructor) say, I can't give him mouth to mouth because I'm pregnant and I can smell the chlorine. Thank God that the paramedics came quickly and got me on oxygen. I had to spend the night in the emergency room on oxygen and the doctor said I was lucky I didn't burn my lungs. Yikes. I will say that the two owners of the gym came to the hospital, stayed and took care of everything. They were really great about the whole thing and I think they cared but I also think they were worried that I might sue. They gave me a few paid days off as well. I wouldn't have sued because it was my fault. Although, you could argue that I wasn't taught how to handle a dangerous chemical and I was a young 21-year-old. But it felt like I was taken care of and it was an accident. Now where was I.

This was kind of the last straw. I had given everything to this club. I had signed up tons of members, keep the members happy, brought in additional revenue with my personal training program, and worked 60-70 hours a week. I had notice for a while that when I looked at my check the 20 hours of personal trainer was almost as much as my 40 hours for the club. It didn't take a rocket scientist to realize that with a few more clients I could make more than my full-time job. With every decision I've ever made in my life I struggled for weeks to make a decision. It's always hard to let go of the sure thing and bet on yourself. Quitting and starting my own business seemed very irresponsible. That's not something you do. You work for some company your whole life, take a lot of crap, and hope you can retire before they fire you and take away your pension. But I have always been a risk taker. Since my grade school days, I made myself do things I wanted to do even if it scared me. I wanted to be good at basketball so I worked constantly at it all summer. And when the next year came around, I was the MVP of the league. I learned at an early age if I believed in myself and worked really hard, I could achieve what I put my mind too. After weeks of toiling, I finally made the decision and I quit my job to start my own personal training business. Now the real work begins. First up, how do I still train my clients at White Rock Athletic Club now that I quit. I tried to talk to the owners about me just training my clients as an independent contractor. Now remember this was at the beginning of the personal training field. It's not like it is today. There was a lot of unknowns, mainly how lucrative it could be for the club. I said we could do an 80/20 split.

Obviously 20% to the club. Now a days the clubs take 70-80 and give the trainer the rest. I'll talk more about this in a later chapter and tell you why the club taking most of the profits is terrible for the personal training industry.  The owners weren't sold on the idea and I think they're pissed that I quit. It wasn't until one of my clients who grew up with one of the owners marched into his office and demanded that they let me stay as a personal trainer. I don't know what she said or did but the next day I was welcome to conduct my new personal training business at the club. Now, what to call my business.

## Chapter Six

## Frazier Fitness

It wasn't a stretch to call my business Frazier Fitness. My last name is Frazier and I was into fitness, so I think I came up with it in five minutes. But I wanted a log line. Something that could easily sum up my new business in one small sentence. I wanted to convey how I felt about the fitness business. That it was more than just working out. It is everything from sleep, to what you eat, to managing your stress. I came up with it in an hour or so. It's the slogan I still use today which is thirty years later. "It's not just a workout, it's a way of life!" Got to say I'm still proud of that log line today. It says everything I want to say with very few words.  I was at my friend's house, Jim. Still don't know why we did this but we got a balloon and tied a piece of paper with the name of my business and log line on it and let it go. I guess it was to be symbolic of launching a new business. In order to do that I needed some seed money to get started. I had enough clients to pay most of my bills but needed just a little more to get cards printed and do a little advertising. Jim, my first home client and friend loaned me

$600 to get through the first few months. That's right it only cost $600 in 1992 to start a business. Not really but I knew nothing of starting a business. I had a high school degree and two years at a performing arts college. But the most important thing I had was heart. I had a determination to make it happen and a 22 years old energy to work my butt off. I really never thought about failing. I only thought about how to make it work. I had ideas that weren't all that complicated. I was going to go to places that other trainers didn't think of to get clients. As an independent trainer I couldn't work at a normal gym. They already had their personal training programs in place and would only pay the trainer maybe 50% if you were lucky. I saw an untapped market at high end apartments that were building fitness rooms and at country clubs that had small fitness rooms. That's in addition to the clients I had at White Rock Athletic Club. I also picked up clients at the Y.M.C.A. and I worked for another trainer at her small gym. Basically, I did anything and everything to get the business going. I worked extremely hard. Probably twelve-to-fourteen-hour days. If I wasn't in a session, I was working on getting clients. As hard as I worked, I have to say that some of it was easy. Much easier than starting over ten years later in Los Angeles. More on that later. I would go into the apartment complex office or country club office and just pitch myself. It was easier because nobody else was doing this at the time. Remember this was the very beginning of personal training going mainstream. I would go in and tell them it would benefit them by providing an instructor as an extra service to their members. Also, I said by providing a trainer you would lesson your liability if someone got hurt on the equipment. Very quickly I had an apartment building and two country clubs allowing me to put up my cards and brochures in their fitness rooms and if you can believe it, I talked them into letting me teach a free class to the members, which they actually paid me, I believe it was $35 for the class. On Tuesday evenings I would teach a class at the apartment complex and on Thursday I would teach one at the country club and then I talked my apartment complex manager into letting me teach a workout class on Monday nights and they took $100 off my rent each month.

I started to get creative with the classes at the country club. I also talked them into letting me write a fitness article in their monthly newsletter. I would write a little paragraph on some topic and then list the four classes for the month. I came up with different focuses for each class, like "Get a slimmer waist".  Knowing what the interest is at a country club, I came up with my most popular class "How to improve your golf game". Wholly crap did I hit on something. Now, I don't know how to play golf but I do know what muscles are involved and what would help improve someone's game. That class was very popular. In fact, one time we had to turn away people because so many people showed up. It was a very small fitness room maybe 400 square feet. It would be full with ten people but sometimes that class would have up to twenty people in the room.  From there I started to get clients. And the more guy's golf games improved the more clients I got. I quickly became "the guy to see" if you wanted your golf game to get better. Remember I'm not teaching golf, I'm teaching fitness and stretching. The more flexible and stronger the mid-section the farther you drive the ball. Sorry to say but it wasn't rocket science. I worked very hard building a fitness business but I have to confess it was kind of easy. What I mean by that is that everything I tried worked. I had a plan I went into the meetings with a lot of unearned confidence and everybody said yes. Maybe not all of them right away but pretty quickly. Remember that this is 1992 and there wasn't a lot of competition in the fitness field especially the way I was doing it. Yes, there were 24-hour fitness and other chain gyms and clubs that had personal training programs but very few independent trainers at that time. When I first started on my own, I worked for another trainer as a contractor and that's when I got my first cell phone, if you want to call it that. Way back in the day "kids" there was a time before cell phones and internet and GPS and stuff like that. It's almost laughable now but the standard Uniform for a trainer was either bicycle shorts or MC hammer pants (for the kids MC Hammer pants were extremely baggy long pants with very colorful prints) and a t-shirt of some kind, and a fanny pack with a beeper. Yes, you read that right. Hopefully I can find some old photos to put into this book so you can see that I was telling the truth. Now that I had my own business and was traveling around, I needed a business number. My pager was my business number but I needed a way to call someone back if I was on the road. The owner of this small personal training gym gave me her old cell phone which was "The Brick" If you're not familiar it is one of the first portable cell phones that came out sometime in the 80's. It was literally the size of a brick with a long thick black antenna. It took 10-12 hours to charge and give you maybe 10–15-minute talking time. Not that you would want to talk on it very long because I think it cost something outrageous like a dollar or two a minute. That's why mainly rich people had cell phones at the time.

It's funny how the mind works but that's about all I remember from my time there. I don't remember the name of the place or the name of the nice lady that gave me a chance or any of the clients that I trained there. I do remember that it was very brief maybe a couple of months and then I moved on. At that time, I had Lakewood Country Club, Dallas Athletic Club, and The Weddington Apartment Complex, and my clients at White Rock.  Still, most of my clients were at White Rock and that's where I spent most of my time mainly during the day. I had three classes I taught at night, Monday at my apartment complex, Tuesday at the Weddington, and Thursday at the DAC (country club). Within six months I was up in running and was making a living. I was able to pay back my friend, Jim within the year. Although, I was making a living I was constantly working on the business. I put money back into the business.  A lot of printing. Remember, back then there was no advertising on line, everything was printed. I printed cards, brochures, t-shirts, whatever it took to get the name out there. My clients were (and still are today) very dedicated to my business. I truly believe, that alone, is the secret to a successful business. Client loyalty! It really just comes down to that. Now getting that, can be tricky. But I never tried to get client's loyalty, I perhaps got their loyalty because I worked hard, had a good attitude, took real interest in my clients and really wanted to help them reach their fitness goals.  I always try to put the client first.

More on that in a later chapter of the success in business.  So now I've been in business for a year and things were going well. But there was no time to take the foot off the pedal. I needed to keep growing, keep advertising. Clients would come and go. Some were what I call, a one off. Basically, someone who would do one maybe two sessions to get started and I wouldn't see them again. I had my core group of clients and then I would fill the rest of the day with one off's. There were always many hours during the middle of the day where I had nothing. Which I would use to do business stuff and workout. The first year I spent so much of my time building a business that I didn't work out all that much. I still workout but not like I was used to doing. Since things were off and running, I decided that I was going to put on some muscle. At the time I was 175 lbs. I was fit but wanted more.  I started working out a lot. My days would consist of training clients in the morning have lunch and workout for three hours. Yes, three hours five to six times a week. It sounds crazy now, but that's what it took. In my early twenties my metabolism was really fast which was great because I could eat anything I wanted and didn't gain weight. But it also made it hard to put on muscle. So now at 23-24 years old I was going to get serious about putting on muscle. I did an hour to an hour and a half of one body part, one hour of cardio, and thirty minutes of ads. I know, crazy. But I was young and had all sorts of energy. Now, I just get tired thinking about what I use to do. One day was chest, one day was back, then legs, then arms, and the fifth day was a combo of all of it. And then I would do other variations like, Chest/Triceps, Back/Biceps, Shoulders/Legs, rest day then repeat. There are a lot of ways to put together a routine depending on what you want to do. But for building muscle that's what I did. Most my client however would do a full body workout two to three times a week.  I never trained body builders, mainly because I wasn't one. If someone wanted that I would refer them to someone that was a body builder. At the time I did train myself like a body builder just without the steroids. The only thing I took was protein power and creatine. Creatine is just a supplement to help in the healing of muscle so you could build muscle faster.  Working out that hard and consistently, it still took over a year to put on 15 lbs. of muscle. And now I was in the best shape of my life. Oh, how I long for those days. Not the work to get there but the level of fitness I was at the time. Next stop, grow Frazier Fitness some more.

# Chapter Seven

## Phase II

About two years into business, I had this desire to be the next "Fitness Guru". I was establishing myself in Dallas as a solid business. I would run into people and they would say they have heard of Frazier Fitness. They could be lying and some probably were but I did do a lot of marketing. My cards were everywhere. I would talk to everybody about what I did. I would leave cards on tables at restaurants, on billboards everywhere. Just promote, promote, promote. And then I made T-shirts that my clients would buy from me and they would promote for me. I would be at White Rock sitting in the corner waiting on a client and someone would come up to me and whisper, "I heard you're the guy". At first, I didn't know what they meant. I would say I don't sell drugs. "No, the guy that can get you fit." This happened a lot. Older gentlemen would say the same thing to me like they heard it in the locker room like it was some big secret.  I kind of got a kick out of it because I found it to be pretty funny. It was if I had the key to everlasting life or something.

To continue to grow the business I had an idea to approach the companies that sold home gym equipment. At the time I didn't realize what a good idea that was. I did what I did in the past and went in with a lot of unearned confidence, had a nice portfolio to give to them and pitched them my idea. The only difference this time was that after they sold and delivered the equipment I would go into the homes and give them a demonstration of the equipment for free. Everybody likes free stuff.  I told them that it might help in the sale of the equipment because some people are afraid of not knowing how to use it so therefore, they are not sure if they should spend the money. I also, told them that if they let me go to the homes, that I could get the client to buy more equipment. Needless to say, it was a slam dunk. I would like to take this time to say that none of that was a lie. Even at 24-25 years old I knew people. Most people don't want to spend a lot of money on something they don't know if they are going to use. And after a while they would get a little bored with the same exercises and I would suggest dumbbells or bands or a fitness ball. All stuff that would benefit them, so I wasn't just up-selling them. I guess in other words I wasn't full of shit. I believed in what I was doing and people could tell. I never thought this was rocket science but I guess not everybody is aware that sometimes you just have to be genuine.

Now that I sold the fitness store on my idea, how do I make money from this. By this time, I truly believed in what I was doing and my skill level as a trainer. I started to do the free demo sessions. It would take 45 minutes to an hour. I would simple just show them how the equipment worked and some standard guidelines for a workout.  I was very enthusiastic and at the end I would tell them I could always come back and set them up on a program and I would give them my card and brochure and answer any question they had. I think it was a good presentation. The only "trick" I used is that I didn't let them do all the exercises. I would show the client how to do it and let them try one or two. I don't think it was a trick because it was mainly for time. I had to be done in an hour to get to the next one. Little did I know almost everybody that I did a demo for signed up for at least one or two sessions and some became lifelong clients.  Over the 30 years of training, I believe my success rate for getting a client from a demo is between 90 and 95%. That is a real stat. I soon realized that I wasn't really selling fitness I was selling myself and I'm thankful that people liked what I was selling. There are tons and tons of trainers. You can get anybody to show you how to workout but it helps a lot if you like who's torturing you. My way of training has always been serious about the work but let's have fun in between sets. Talk, laugh, and distract from the pain of working out. To be honest very few people like working out. Yes, they might like how it makes them feel and the results of a fitter body but the actually doing of it most could care less. In fact, if there was any way that someone could pay me to work out for them and they get the results I would be a millionaire many times over. Also, I always make sure that the client comes first. The relationship between trainer and client can become a close one. After all it is called "personal" training. The only problem with that is that the trainer always has to keep in mind that they are being paid to be there and it's about the client. I've seen other trainers fall in the trap of getting close to clients and the clients become the therapist for the trainer. It's OK to share. My clients know tons about me. I just make sure that I'm not "dumping on them". If they want to dump on me all their troubles (which a lot have over the years) that's OK. When you work out it releases a lot of things stored in the body. I've had clients break down and cry during a workout. I've had clients confess very personal things to me. The mind and body are connected and, in some ways, I feel like I'm a therapist as well. Just like a bartender or hair stylist is a "therapist". I'm not saying I'm a therapist! My therapist would be upset if I said I was one.

Recently, I was having a huge issue on the way to my client's house. I was very upset and found it very hard to focus. When I got there, I asked if I could be there as a friend because I really needed to bounce something off someone before I had to face it.  They were very kind and understanding and sat and talked with me for the next few hours. Now they have also become friends of mine. I think it was fine in that one case but the trick is not to let that happen all the time. If I did that all the time or even somewhat often it wouldn't be OK. But it did show that I'm not a robot and that I'm human.

In the growth of Frazier Fitness, I started to go to these fitness conventions that would take place in New York, Miami, and one was in Dallas. You would go and meet other people in the fitness industry, take classes to keep your certification up to date, and then socialize. It's funny over the years I realized that people in the fitness industry can be the biggest "partiers" of them all. I guess it is work hard and play hard. Or we were all young and that's just what you do.

At one of the conventions in New York I took a class. It was an aerobics class and I don't remember why I took it, maybe it was all that available, but that class was taught by a famous fitness woman. She had fitness videos and I believe she was one of the "Buns of Steel" video instructors. If you don't know what that is, it was a popular fitness videos in the 80's. Anyway, I thought she was one of the most beautiful things I have ever seen. She was kind and sweet while she taught which made her even more beautiful. I don't know if I did the moves in the class or if I stood there staring the whole time.

But after the class I knew I had to meet her. Believe it or not after the class she was mobbed. I did get to meet her for a brief second but that wasn't enough for me. I liked her but I also thought I could learn from her. After all she was doing what I wanted to do which was to be a fitness guru. I decided to write her. I think I faxed her a letter because I thought that might get her attention. (Oh yeah, faxing is what we did before email was invented) At the time I was merely trying to approach her as a professional.  I considered her way out of my league. I don't remember exactly what I wrote but something got her attention because she wrote back. It was very sweet what she said and we began writing each other and that turned into phone calls. I mean epic three-hour phone calls. She lived in Miami and I was in Dallas which is one hour difference. We would stay up to midnight (her 1:00 am) ever though we both had to get up early. It quickly went from professional to personal to a very deep connection. She encouraged my pursuit to be the next fitness guru. I was quickly falling in love and I think she was too. It all came to a head about six months later when she was going to be in New York and asked if I could get away for the weekend. The only problem, I was getting my wisdom teeth out on that Friday. On top of that my best friend and his wife were in New York and he said I could stay with them. At the time this low-end airline was offering $99 flights to Newark and you could just take the bus to New York City. I had taken the weekend to recover from getting my wisdom teeth out. So, what was stopping me. Probably not the wisest (Pun intended) decision but I booked the flight and told her I would meet her there. Of course, my surgery was more complicated than it was supposed to be. My wisdom teeth were impacted and the surgery took twice as long. So long I actually woke up in the middle of it. After it was over a friend drove me home and I immediately started to pack. Now I'm in no shape to be getting on a plane the next day but I thought I could rest that night and be fine the next day. Love will make you do crazy things. I get up and get on the plane. The whole time on the plane I'm icing my face. Pain be damned I need to be with this woman. I will say looking back on that weekend it still is one of the best weekends I have ever had. It was something out of a dream or movie. We went to the top of the Empire State building, took a carriage ride around central park (it was November and cold so we snuggled together under a big red blanket), and had romantic dinners. I never needed to stay with my friend, if you know what I mean. Just about a perfect weekend as you can have. It was time to go and we had to part. I felt like I could have just floated back to Dallas. But what they don't cover in romantic movies is reality. Two days later I got dry sockets where my wisdom teeth were taking out. Dry sockets are basically nerves that are exposed to the open air, so when you breath in and the air hits the nerve, you want to die. Or it feels like you are going to die. I went to the dentist immediately and they pack the holes with something that looks like chewing tobacco that is soaked in Novocain. Pain instantly gone. I never told the dentist about my trip. He says it just happens to some people but I'm pretty sure it's because I got on a plane. As painful as it was, I wouldn't have done anything differently. Life is about experiences and that's one experience that was worth it. As for the relationship, well like most long distant relationships it didn't work out. We tried for six months or so and tried to be friends after that but eventually it faded away. She still holds a special place in my heart and I hope she is well.

In the mean time I was steadily growing Frazier Fitness and started to get so busy that I needed to add some trainers. Only as part time contactors but it was moving in the right direction. The only problem, most people wanted me and only me. If I couldn't convince them to go with one of my trainers then I would put them on a waiting list until I had an opening. Which is crazy to think about now. But at the time I built a reputation with a lot of hard work. Things are going well after four almost five years of building the business, I mean what could go wrong. But things were about to change for the rest of my life.

## Chapter Eight

## The Diagnosis

Things seemed to be going along well. The business was successful and I wasn't having to hustle as much to get business. For the last almost five years I have been beating the pavement and now things were coming to me. Referrals and constant work from the home gym stores was keeping me busy and allowing me to add trainers as contract workers. I was still working out really hard to "practice what I was preaching".  But that's when things started to go wrong. I was lifting heavy at the time. I was squatting around 350 lbs. which for my size was a lot. Not a power lifter but not bad for 26 years old.  I started noticing that after leg day my back would go out. Specifically, the S.I. joint (the little ball like thing next to your tailbone). I would go to my friend who was a physical therapist and he would "put them back in". This started to happen every week. I didn't know why. I tried to not lift as heavy but it would still happen. I also started to feel more tired than usual. Needing to take a nap, sleep more at night. Not like me I had energy for days. On one trip to the physical therapist, he happens to poke around and pushed on my lower abdomen. I jumped in pain and ask what the hell was that. He said it was my lymph nodes and they were extremely swollen. He didn't know what was causing it but maybe there was a connection.  Over the next weeks it was hard to workout and I was getting more fatigue by the day. Then worse stuff started to happen. How should I put this? I couldn't keep anything down. Or should I say everything I ate went right through me. I started cutting stuff out like milk or any dairy. Maybe I have become allergenic to some type of food. I tried everything. By the end I was eating tuna out of the can and raw vegetables. But I still couldn't keep anything down. I began to get weaker and weaker. I could barely workout. I was tried all the time and in pain. Doctor appointment after doctor appointment nobody could find anything. One doctor even said it was in my head. At this point I had lost 20 lbs. so how could it be in my head. I didn't have much fat so the 20 lbs. was muscle and I was mal nourished so I started to get that sunken in look. They finally did a colonoscopy or the less evasive sigmoidoscopy. They found nothing. I started to think I was going crazy. After many months of this I finally got a break. A friend of mine from the gym who was a doctor was asking me about what was going on. I told him everything and then he asked me to get up and walk down the hall. He stood behind me and watched me walk. He said my gate was off and he referred me to a friend who was a specialist. The doctor took x-rays, blood, and a full exam. A week later I go back and he had a diagnosis. He said I had an arthritic condition called ankylosing spondylitis or A.S. for short. Basically, it is arthritis of the spine and hips that causes the spine to swell and can pinch the nerves and cause the muscles to get stiff. Ultimately, your spine could fuse together. If it sounds like it sucks, it really really does. There is no cure and back in the 90's there was very little treatment. The doctor said just make sure you stand up straight so when the spine fuses at least you won't be humped over. Oh great, thanks. I was in some way glad I had a diagnosis but there wasn't a damn thing I could do about it. It was at the time a very difficult thing to diagnose and there was very little know about it. That doctor sent me to an arthritis doctor and I would do physical therapy. I go to the arthritis specialist and I was the youngest person there by 50 years. He decided to put me on this drug which maybe helped because I could start to keep food down. The only problem the drug made me really sleepy. I fell asleep at the wheel and almost crashed my car so I stopped taking that drug. After six months I go see the doctor and he wants to try a different drug. I asked why and he really didn't have a good answer and that's when it hit me, I was a guinea pig. Every six months they would try me on a different medication and see how I do. I didn't feel like the drugs really helped that much so I stopped taking them. I would have to find another way.

I didn't know what that would be. I knew that I couldn't lift heavy weights anymore so I started to do lighter weight more reps' kind of workout and only did weights four times a week instead of 5-6 times. I started doing a lot more stretching and cardio. The cardio seemed to help if I was stiff. When I wasn't having a "flare-up" back then I would mostly be fine. Early on flare-ups would occur maybe four times a year. Some lasting weeks and some of the worse ones would last up to three months. I would get massages, go to the chiropractor, do acupuncture, and get in the steam room to help loosen me up. Now I'm not going to lie the pain was and is bad. But in some ways, I can take that more than the fatigue. There are times during flare-ups that I would get up train my clients and go home and nap then get up and train some more clients nap again off and on all day. There were some days, probably more than I would like to admit, that I would just take a sick day and sleep. There were times where I thought I would just sleep my life away. Even when I was awake, I wasn't myself. I still would "put on a good face" when I was with my clients but I didn't have the same energy that I use to have. Fortunately, my business didn't seem to suffer but I was wearing down.

When you are first diagnosed with a disease (I would like to point out that the word disease is dis /ease meaning not at ease) you don't know what to do. Do I keep it to myself, do I tell everybody, what do I say? At the time I was diagnosed I was 27 years old which is kind of young to be told that you have a lifelong disease, so it felt like a big deal to me. I decided to tell family and close friends and a few very close clients. After all I could hide most the symptoms so maybe only a few people needed to know. Although I would do things differently now, I would sit down with a friend or friends and make it out to be this big announcement and sadly tell them the news. I think I did it that way because I really didn't understand what I was diagnosed with. They were still a lot I didn't know. After I told the people I wanted to tell, I felt weird about it. I didn't know if I wanted sympathy or encouragement or what. I didn't quit get the reaction from my family that I thought. It was kind of not a reaction at all. It was as if I was making it up. So, I decided not to talk about it too much to the point that most friends and family forgot about it. Like I said I could hide it pretty well back then. I didn't walk noticeably different and I lived alone so no one knew all the naps I took and most the time I felt OK so maybe I shouldn't talk about it?

The one symptom I didn't bring up is depression. Don't worry I'm going to cover that more in a later chapter but it bares mentioning now. The one thing the diagnoses did was reevaluate my life. I had worked so hard for the past five years building the business I didn't stop and ask myself if I was happy. I got so caught up into building a fitness empire I forgot why I started it in the first place. What I'm about to say doesn't take away my passion and dedication to fitness and my clients. But when I first started, I thought it would be a good way to make good money so I could spend the rest of my time pursuing an acting career. It had been six years since the performing arts program. Most students from my class moved to New York to give it ago and my best friend Scott, started singing on cruise ships right away. I got caught up into building a business, and kind of forgot about my dream. I remember the day it hit me like a ton of bricks. I had just finished with a client at Lakewood Country Club and was having brunch at Cafe Brazil by myself and started wondering why I was unhappy. I mean my business was successful, it had been several months since my diagnoses and I had accepted it, not thrilled obviously but trying to deal with it. And then it hit me. ACTING! It was almost like a little voice from somewhere shouted it at me. All of a sudden, I knew what I had to do, get back into the game, but how. It is funny how something like a bad diagnosis makes you start to rethink things. I started wondering if the A.S. would progress to the point that I couldn't be a trainer.  I just didn't know what was

going to happen but I did know I wasn't completely fulfilled so
I had to do something about it. That discovery happened
towards the end of the year so I decided that in the new year I
would do something I hadn't done, take time off.  In the past I
would take vacation and be gone for a week but I never took
two full weeks off. In February I took two weeks, one week in
town and one week in New York to see my friend Anne. I
wanted to go to New York to see if maybe I should move there
for acting. I think I was still reeling from my diagnoses from six
months earlier and needed to sort things out in my head. It
was a great trip. Anne had to work so I would go and do stuff
during the day and we would hang out at night. My main
reason to go to New York was to meet my favorite actress
Sarah Jessica Parker. I for some reason thought if I meet her, I
would know if I should pursue acting. I know, totally nuts but I
had a plan. Before I left, I bought a ticket to a Broadway show
"The Princess and the Pea" which Miss Parker was staring in
at the time. I wrote a perfectly drafted letter (I say perfectly
because I went through several drafts so I wouldn't come
across as a stalker) and I was going to buy flowers and put the
letter with it. I went to the theatre early to drop them off at
the stage door. Farfetched I know but you have to have a
plan. Anne couldn't afford a ticket to the show and with
taking two weeks and traveling I really couldn't afford two
tickets so the plan was for me to go to the show and Anne

would meet me after for drinks. So off I go early to the show. I stopped and bought a half dozen red roses that were really amazing. Really some of the most beautiful roses I had ever seen. Why a half dozen you might ask, they were really expensive. But got to say worth it. So, I put the letter with the flowers and off to the theatre I went. It was cold and snowing but very beautiful. I was so happy I was going to see Sarah Jessica in a live show. I had a great seat since I was by myself. It was the third row I remember. I had no idea what was going to happen when I went to the stage door with the flowers but like always, I went up to the door with that unearned confidence. There was this big guy outside the door and I went up to him and said "I have flowers for Miss Parker" Without missing a beat he opened the door. I walked in like I belonged and then there was another big guy seated there. I said again, I have flowers for Miss Parker. He said I can take them and then I said something stupid like I could bring them to her dressing room. He said no and that he would take them and if there was anything to sign. Then it hit me they thought I was a delivery guy. I did have black pants and a black leather jacket. I quickly said no there was nothing to sign and I turned to exit. Unbelievably right then as I'm about to get to the door guess who enters. Yeah, one guess, Sarah Jessica Parker.  And we actually ran into each other. If it was a movie, it would have been what they call a meet-cute. She looked up at me and without recognizing me the first thing she said is "you can't be in here". I don't know how I really keep it together. I smiled and said calmly "I was just dropping off flowers for you." The guy behind me said something like "he cool" and then she relaxed. I said have a great show and left. I couldn't believe what had just happened and that I totally keep my cool. It wasn't totally by accident. With my limited acting knowledge, I know that a call time before a show is usually two hours and that's right when I was there. I also, knew that Sarah was a professional and would probably be on time. I was right but also lucky. Thirty seconds either way and I wouldn't have literally run into her. But after the show it even gets better. The show was great and Sarah (I can call her that because we just meet and we're on a first name basis) was amazing in the show. After the show I was in front of the theatre waiting for my friend and I noticed some people lining up around the stage door. Obviously, they were waiting for Sarah to come out, so I walked near where everybody was waiting. I stood back because there were little girls wanting autographs and sure enough, she came out and signed autographs and was very gracious. I was on the fence if I should make my way over and say "great show" or something like that when the strangest thing happened. Sarah looked up and recognized me. She immediately said those were such beautiful flowers and we started talking. She had a car and driver waiting for her but she seemed willing to stand there and talk. I know I said something like great show but otherwise I can't remember what was said but it did go on for several minutes. I remember thinking I don't know how long I can play it cool so I said something like I needed to go and I walked away with her standing there. I left so abruptly that I could feel that she was staring at the back of my head. I fought the instinct of turning around and keep on walking. Now remember I'm supposed to meet my friend in front of the theatre so I had to walk down the street and around the corner and wait until her car drove away. It went about as well as it could at the time. Now twenty-five years later I would have been able to carry on a conversation better but in my defense Sarah Jessica Parker was the first famous person I had ever engaged in conversation. I never in my wildest dreams would have thought that I would get to meet her and have a conversation. I don't think she will ever know how important it was to me that she was kind and friendly. It left me with such a great feeling that I could do anything. Right or wrong I took it as a sign that I should get back into acting. I know it still doesn't make since but Sarah talking to me made me thing that I belonged in the acting world. After a great trip I got back to Dallas and decided to get back into acting. I started taking an acting class at a place called S.T.A.G.E. It's an acronym but I forgot what it stands for. Gail was my first acting teacher for theatrical acting (TV and film). I learned so much from her. I started meeting people and found out about a casting director workshop. Wow, the person that cast you in commercials and TV shows and films. There were only four people in the workshop and I befriended another actor. We stayed in touch and he asked me to do a showcase in front of a crowd of other actors, directors and agents. I was nervous but excited and we did a scene that the casting director gave us in the workshop called "The Fly". One of the funniest scenes I've ever seen to this day.  Basically, I play a guy who really believes he is a fly and has a conversation with a stranger about what his purpose is in life. We worked very hard to make this perfect and it was. Not only did we get the biggest laughs we won best scene of the night. I didn't know this but my scene partner's agent came and was very complementary of my performance. She wanted to sign my on the spot. I had one other agent interested but I wanted to go with someone that was excited about me, so I signed with my first real agent at the age of 27. Now acting in Dallas, Texas is way different than acting in Los Angeles. At best I would have one or two auditions a month. Sometimes it would be months before another audition would come. And let me tell you I was bad at auditioning. Maybe the worse. There is just something so nerve racking about the process, plus I was new to it. It is a terrible process, especially nonprofessional auditions. Which was mainly all I went out for early on. Sometimes it would take hours just to audition for two sentences. Since they were non-union auditions, they could take as long as they wanted. Union auditions have to go by union rules and if they make an actor wait too long you have to start paying them. Not that anybody I have met got paid for waiting in an audition but I have heard that it does happen on a rare occasion. Mainly, the early years of acting was mainly acting classes and some local theatre and an occasional audition for a commercial, an industrial (that's a video made for companies to show their employees) or an independent film. Most of my days were spent on Frazier Fitness. Training my clients, marketing, working out and growing the business.

Looking back, it seems that I would have three or four flare ups with the A.S. a year. Back then most of the time I would be OK. I would always have some pain but if I had to assign a number value, I would say I was always at a three and during flare-ups anywhere between an eight and really bad ones so far off the charts I couldn't even tell you. So, what's a flare-up? I would say it's an extended period of time with high inflammation in my body that is very painful and completely exhausting. They start out the same. Extreme fatigue and diarrhea. Why diarrhea? I don't really know but my best guess from research is the swelling in my low back presses on the nerves that control the intestines. Don't quote me on that, I'm not a doctor. Then the stiffness sets in which makes it hard to stand up straight, or bend over, or twist, sit too long, stand too long, or do almost anything. And lastly the pain in the spine. It is sore to the touch and just throbs all day long. I usual describe it as a knife being jammed into my spine. And no that's not an exaggeration. It can be excruciating at times. But oddly the pain is not the worst thing about it. It is the fatigue. Sounds crazy but somehow, I am able to accept the pain and put it in the back of my mind, most of the time. Most people with chronic pain knows what I'm talking about. My friend Jim, early on thought I had narcolepsy because every time I would sit down, I would fall asleep. I struggled to stay awake while I was driving. I nodded off so much it's a miracle I didn't have a huge car accident. It's the fatigue that is really hard to comprehend. If you have had the flu really bad and you are so sick that all you can do is sleep, it's kind of like that. Remember, I'm working 12-14 hours a day. Not straight through but sometimes I would start training at 6 a.m. and finish at 8 p.m. Fortunately, I would have several hours during the day that I could take a nap. During times of flare-ups, I wouldn't do much except train a client and then go home and sleep. Then I would get up and train the next client and then go back to sleep. And on and on until the flare-up would pass. Exercise was either light or nonexistent during that time. I do remember I could go six months between flare-ups and feel reasonably OK during that time. But as the years went on the flare-ups would increase in frequency and intensity. I didn't know then but the worse was still to come.

Chapter Nine

Moving Time

After ten years of building Frazier Fitness, I decided to follow my dream of acting and move to Los Angeles. I had been thinking about it for a few years and even made two trips to Los Angeles to get the lay of the land. I had always heard to do as much acting work in your hometown before moving to Los Angeles. Like so many other people I believe that 9/11 had a lot to do with my decision to move. September 11, 2001 changed everything. I really started to look at my life and try to figure out what I really wanted to do. As the year started in 2002, I had decided that I would move to Los Angeles in 2003. It gave me a year to decide what to do with my business, to do as much acting work in Dallas before I moved, and to pay off debt and save as much money as I could. It was hard to save when most of my money would go back into my business that I was creating. Oddly after working so hard to build a business, I was willing to give it all up on a dream. At that time, I had been acting for four years. I booked some regional commercials, (regional means the commercial is only shown in that part of the country.) Local commercials (only shown in the Dallas market) and industrials (things that are shot for companies to show in house to their employees.) and a few independent films (films shot by individuals on a shoestring budget). My most memorable acting jobs where a local commercial I did for a fast-food chain Golden Chic. Kind of like Chic-fil-a. I was in the commercial with Jay Novacek, a just retired tight-end for the Dallas Cowboys. I was a little star stuck but he was such a nice guy that I felt relaxed very quickly and we had a great day shooting the commercial. Another thing I did which was probably the biggest thing I did was for the American Red Cross. It was the videos they use in teaching CPR and first aid. It was a big project and I was cast in two different parts. I played a dad around a pool with his child. If I remember correctly, it was about pool safety. But the second was my starring role as "Choking Ken". The guy that chokes at a restaurant and the waiter gives me the Heimlich. On the day I'm sitting in a fake restaurant in a warehouse that was very dusty. I'm sitting at a table with my "wife" and eating Mexican food. The food was real and I would take a bite and then hold the food in my mouth and after he pretends to give me the Heimlich, I would spit the food out of my mouth and onto the floor and some poor P.A. would have to pick up the food I spit out over and over again. I don't know how many times we did the take but it was more than five and less than ten. On one of the takes I put the food in my mouth and as I was pretending to choke, I sucked in too much air and the food got stuck in my throat. (I know the irony) Now I was choking but not to the point that I needed the Heimlich but the funny thing was I was making the sign for choking which is two hands around your throat. For a minute no one knew I was really choking but I knew I could cough it up. In order to let everybody know that it was real I walked off set and finally coughed it up onto the floor and yes that poor P.A. had to clean it up as well. The medic came over and it became a big deal which was just so embarrassing to me at the time. I just wanted to do a good job and now I'm the idiot that really choked when I was pretending to choke. It's hilarious now and a great story to tell but at the time I was mortified. We did go back and shoot more takes of me choking so in the end I was very professional. That video was used for years in CPR and first aid classes. I had more friends and family see that then just about anything I have every done. As I write this, I had some old VHS Tapes transferred over to digital form and my old demo reel was one of the tapes. I couldn't believe it but I still have footage of the Golden Chic commercial, the CPR video, and few other things I had forgotten about. These VHS tapes were over 22 years old and the quality wasn't great but I still have footage. Sometimes it's good to go down memory lane. It's not always as we remember but, in this case, it was pretty close. I have definitely gotten better as an actor. Now, were was I, oh yes moving. I don't know if you can plan a trip in any more details. I had charts and lists, who to tell when. Very detailed about the move, maybe a little OCD about it. It was the biggest decision of my life and the only way I was going to feel good about it is if I had it planned to the very last detail. There are two types of people, ones that can just pick up and move across the country and ones that stay put and are born and die in the same town. I'm more of the latter forcing myself to be the former. I was getting things done but I still didn't know what to do with the business. Pieces of the puzzle were falling into place except Frazier Fitness. I knew that the business had value I just didn't know how to quantify it. Then one day about six months before the move a friend called me to give his buddy some advice. He was a trainer at a gym and was giving most of what he was making to the gym which is all too common. I called Jeff and started to give him advice on the personal training business. I surprised myself on how much knowledge about training I had accumulated. Stupidly, it didn't dawn on me to see if Jeff was interested in Frazier Fitness until the end of the conversation. But we had made plans to have lunch and talk more about it. Over the next few weeks, I realized that this was a perfect fit. Only thing to do was tell my clients and get Jeff trained in the "Frazier Fitness" way. That's kind of a joke but I did want him to shadow me just to see what the clients were doing and how I worked with them. I knew in order for him to be able to maintain the clients he couldn't do things drastically different or the clients might not stay. Nobody likes change so the easier I could make the transition, the better it would be for everybody. The only thing left for me to do was book one more acting job, to help me know I was doing the right thing. I guess I needed a sign. And the sign came with a movie called "Ocean Front Property". It was late summer and I had gotten a cold. Nothing too bad but I had a low fever and congestion. I had already gone in for the first audition for the role of Stan and this was the call-back. (A call-back is a second audition which means it's down to just a few actors) I even called the director and asked if I could come another day because I was sick. He said that this was the only day for call-backs so I got my shit together and went to the audition. In Dallas the acting community was pretty small so I usually knew everybody at the auditions. And of course, the one guy that I always went up against was there for the same part. I was so sick that I really didn't care. I mean I wanted the part but I was too sick to care too much which is the real secret to acting. More on that later. The director, Joe, was very nice and ask everybody if it was OK for me to go first because I was sick. I'm over there coughing in the corner and everybody was like, yeah get this guy out of here. Little did I know that Joe really wanted me for the part but had already cast my wife, so he just wanted to make sure the chemistry was right.

In Hollywood they call it a screen test. He brought in a few other actors to compare the difference. I don't really remember the audition but I do remember thinking that I did pretty well. I think it was the next day that I got the call that I got the part. It was a paying film which was a big deal. Most independent films don't pay or pay very little. I got "my sign" that I should move to Los Angeles. The film was shot in late September early October. It was about two and a half weeks which is very short period of time to shoot a movie (most movies take three to six months and some can take up to 18 months) Before we went to Galveston to shoot, the financial backer pulled out but we decided as a group that we would still do it and not get paid. It was a good group of people and a good project that doesn't come along too often. That was the best decision we made because it was one of the best times I have ever had on set. They call it a labor of love because that was what it was. Just because something is fun doesn't mean it isn't hard work. As actors if we weren't in the shot, we were working behind the camera as part of the crew. We shot and lived in a beach house in Galveston Texas. It was hot and humid and full of mosquitos. Most days were 16 hours. The longest day, I will never forget. We started at 8:00 am and worked until 7:00pm had dinner and went back to work from 8:00pm until 7:am the next day, IN THE OCEAN.

Yes, the night shoot was in the ocean. And as hot as it was during the day it was pretty cold at night especially in the ocean. As hard as that was it was extremely rewarding to know that we could do that. When they say "suffer for your art" I know exactly what that means.

As great as that project was it was over very quickly and now, I was faced with telling my clients that I was moving to LA LA Land. This was going to be a very difficult task.

Chapter Ten

The Move

As I started to tell clients I started with my longest-term clients. Some had been with me for over 10 years. It was very difficult to tell them because I had grown very close to a lot of my clients. Some of my clients broke down in tears when I told him I was moving. It was very moving that they had liked me that much that they would be sad to see me go. Most clients took it in stride but made it very clear that I would be missed. And although they were sad that I was leaving they were happy that I was pursuing my dreams of being an actor. By the end of 2002 I had told all my clients, friends, and family that as of 2003 I would be moving to Los Angeles. As I said before this is a very hard decision and very unlike something I would do. Most of my friends and family never moved away from Dallas. I think that's normal for most people to grow up and live in the same town. Other people have no problem picking up and moving many times in their life. Although, I had traveled quite a bit it was still very scary to pick up and move away from everything I had ever known. As scary as it was it was equally exciting to embark on a new adventure. I had decided to work through the end of the year of 2002 and Jeff would take over in January 2003 but I would not leave Dallas until the end of January to give me three weeks to help in the transition of Frazier Fitness. Also, it gave me time to pack and say goodbye to friends and family. It's funny but I think I had at least three going away parties. One was a big party that I invited everybody I ever knew and the other was a small dinner party with close friends. I still remember that dinner party and how special it was that my closest friends gathered to wish me well and send me off. I didn't know then that saying goodbye would change the dynamics of my friendships forever. Some friends at that dinner I've even gotten closer to over the years and some have faded away a little bit. It's funny how life can change on you. But I still consider them friends regardless of how much time is past.

It was getting close to the move date I believe it was the 23rd, January 2003. The moving company was coming in the morning to pack everything up and put in storage until I had a place that I was going to live. All of my important stuff I packed in my Jeep Cherokee. The moving company finished by 2 PM which was longer than I thought it would take. The goal was to get on the road and be in Amarillo for my first night. Dallas to Amarillo is about a 6 Hour drive so I arrived about 8 PM. Through the whole trip I mainly stayed at Motel 6 because they allowed dogs for just a few extra dollars a night. The trip itself was very exciting I have never taken a road trip across the country are half the country. I wanted to take my time to see places along the way. From Amarillo I drove to Santa Fe New Mexico which only took four hours so I had a half a day in Santa Fe. It was fun but it would've been better had it been with somebody. I couldn't do a lot because I had Lucy, my dog with me and I didn't want to leave her too long in the motel.

From Santa Fe I went to see the Grand Canyon. That was the longest day I believe it took me 10 hours and I got there by sunset to see the Grand Canyon. I have a great photo of me and my dog Lucy at sunset over the Grand Canyon. This was the only hotel that Lucy couldn't stay with me but they had a dog kennel where she had to stay. I felt bad but it was just for the night I had no other choice as it was dark. I got to spend some time at the Grand Canyon the next day and then we got on the road to Vegas.  I saw the Hoover dam on my way to Henderson Nevada to stay with my friend Scott. The plan was to stay a few days in Vegas and then Scott and I would drive to LA to find an apartment. The drive from Las Vegas to Los Angeles is about 4 to 4 ½ hours. I had done some research online about places to look for based on price. In 2003 you couldn't do as much online as you can now. But we did have a few places to look at. It was shocking what you got for the price, or should I say what you didn't get for the price. The areas that I can afford weren't necessarily the best areas in LA but it was affordable so I picked a place in Van Nuys California. I signed the lease that started February 1, so Scott and I went back to Vegas for about a week. I called the moving company and timed my stuff to be delivered on the first and I would drive to Los Angeles by myself.  The one bedroom was okay but was older and had a lot of issues that I didn't see at the time. Also, I didn't know that there were drug dealers and other criminals in the building. One time I woke up to the ATF knocking on one of my neighbor's door at seven in the morning. That kind of clued me in that I wasn't in the best place. The first month I moved in it rained almost every day in February. So much rain in fact that the walkway above my apartment held too much water so the water started coming down inside my apartment. It looked like it was raining inside my window because the water was running down the window inside my place like one of those fake waterfalls. It flooded the carpets and I had to move all my electronics before they got ruined. So, I was off to a good start in LA. I tried to hit the ground running and got my place set up in about a week. I immediately tried to get work as a personal trainer and at the same time got head shots done for my acting and started signing up for acting classes and workshops. It was very difficult to get started as a trainer in

Los Angeles. I didn't realize at the time but every actor was also a personal trainer. It makes sense because it's a business that's flexible and allows you to be able to audition during the day but I didn't realize how tough the competition would be. All the marketing that I used in Dallas did not work in Los Angeles. I went to country clubs, apartment complexes, and personal training gyms and there were no openings whatsoever. No one was impressed with my 10 years of experience as a personal trainer. I had to prove myself all over again. I finally found the gym that would feed me clients but I had to pay a gym rent of about $300 a month but I had no clients. It was very inexpensive to join this gym so it didn't attract a lot of people that could afford a personal trainer. The deal was the owner would send me names and numbers of the new members and I would give them a free session to try to get business. I remember the first week I gave over 40 hours of free training with no one signing up. I had to make the personal training fee very low in order to attract clients. It took over a month to get just a few clients but it was a start. I also went to another personal training gym but they didn't have any clients for me. I stayed in touch with them and volunteered to help with the Special Olympics kids that they were working with, for free of course. But that got me to prove myself to them and slowly they started giving me clients. I was only making a portion of the personal training fee but it was fair because they were feeding me clients. At the six-month mark I had some clients and was making some money but not enough to live on. Since I still owned Frazier fitness in Dallas, I was making 30% of what the business was pulling in and I was also still running things on my end. I called on clients and handled all the finances but it only took a few hours a week. About at the six-month mark Jeff wanted to buy the business. I understood the hesitancy of buying the business when I first moved. He saw the value in having the whole business after the six-month mark. We made an arrangement that he would pay me 30% of the business for the next year and a half and then the business would be his free and clear. It was a win-win for both of us because he didn't have the money to buy me out all at once and he still had me consulting for another year and a half to help him build up the business. It might be the only personal training business ever sold without having any equipment. But the client list and the Frazier Fitness name that I built over ten years had value. I had worked extremely hard to build a successful business and I was very glad that I could pass it on and see it continue. Now 20 years later Jeff still trains some of the same clients that I had and also has built the business bigger and better. I hope I had some impact on helping him succeed. But he put in the work to build up what is now called Paramount Fitness. It felt good to be able to leave my clients that I cared for so much in good hands instead of just leaving them on their own. I built a business to make a living but also to help people. I had amazing clients in Dallas and I'm proud of the fact that I'm still in touch with a lot of them today. What most people in the fitness business didn't realize is that client loyalty is everything. My clients would've done anything for me and I would've done the same. If someone wants to know how to have success in the personal training world it is to care for your clients. Knowing the anatomy, biomechanics, weightlifting exercises, and stretches are just a small part of having a personal training business. Showing up on time, being consistent with your client's workout times is also very important. But showing your heart and soul is what I think is the biggest part of any business. Working hard is a given but going above and beyond for your clients is where the success lies. It is a fine line to care about your clients and to be friends with them but still remembering the job at hand, first and foremost. Where a lot of trainers go wrong is that they get too close to their client and  the session becomes all about the trainer. It's okay to confide in your clients and to share with them as long as you remember it's about them first. It's a hard line to straddle but I believe I've done it pretty well for most of my career. Not that I haven't made some mistakes but overall, I tried always to remember, the client first. If there's something I can share about my own life that can benefit my client I will share that. Every client has a different motivation about working out, it's the trainer's job to figure out how to best facilitate a workout. For example, some clients want to know everything we're doing and why. And there are other clients that don't care anything about the workout and they just want me to put them through their paces because it's good for them. Knowing the difference is very important. Some clients have different abilities, flexibilities and understanding of their physical body. As much as I try to have a client do an exercise with perfect form sometimes you have to settle for the form that they can do best. It might not be the best form but as long as they're not hurting themselves than you have to let it go sometimes. A personal trainer has to be a people person and has to really understand the different types of people they will come in contact with. It would be great to only find clients that you get along with but that's not how the business world works. So, you have to find a way to work with different types of people. It's something they say in the acting world; "know your audience", this applies to personal training. Know the person that you're training. Over the years I've been able to figure it out in a very, very short period of time sometimes within the first few minutes of meeting someone. If you have different political views, avoid that conversation because it is not important in order to do your job. As a trainer you always want to find common ground with whom you're working with. There is no way over the course of time to only speak about working out. To be honest there is only so much that can be said about working out. Once you've covered the correct form on exercises, explaining all the exercises, talking about nutrition, and how much cardiovascular exercise a client should do, there's not much left to talk about. I have been very fortunate in my career to have very long-term clients. More times than not when I start with a new client, they become a client for very long time if not for life. Although some clients come and go, I found that I can bring something to the table that keeps clients wanting me to come back. And over the years I've realized that is the personal part of personal training not the training part that they have me come back for. It pays to be kind and thoughtful and interested and engaged. I believe that my clients can see the sincerity within me to want to help them. It seems like a no-brainer but I've seen trainers not understand this concept. Client care is the most important thing in retaining a client. All the knowledge in the world won't help, if you don't know how to convey that knowledge in a way in which the client can understand. I think being a personal trainer isn't for everybody. You need to have a certain aptitude for wanting to help people. Also, being an independent personal trainer can have its ups and downs. If the economy is good the business can be good and when the economy is bad to be very bad for business. I've never kid myself that I am a luxury item. No matter how much a client likes me, I will be one of first things to go if a client's finances change. One of the mistakes I've made in my career as a personal trainer is not advertising when I'm busy. My excuse was I was busy and business is fine so why continue to advertise but all it takes is losing a couple clients and I can be financially hurting. And it wasn't easy to just replace those clients, it took time. Advertising is not instantaneous, it's something that has to be done consistently. But of course, word-of-mouth is always the best source of new clients. Unfortunately, I've run into times where my current clientele doesn't really have anybody they can refer. In Los Angeles, location is everything. My clients might have friends that could live geographically close but it could take an hour and a half to get to their house. I found it difficult to get referrals within a certain mile radius. When I was a personal trainer in Dallas Texas at the time, I could get almost anywhere in Dallas within 30 minutes. I know that has changed now but when I first started, Dallas wasn't as big as it is today. In order to have your own personal training business you have to be the trainer, the marketing person, the person that does the finances and everything in between. It can be very rewarding to see the fruits of your labor. But sometimes over time it gets hard to continue to reinvent the wheel over and over again. I know some people reading this right now think it's great to have your own business, to be your own boss, to do what you want but the grass is always greener. Being a business owner there's no paid vacation, no 401K, your tax rate is higher, no paid sick days, and what I find to be the hardest thing is you never know how much money you're going to make every week or every month. Over the years most of my anxiety has come from not knowing how much money I'm going to make every month. I always know what my bills will come to every month, I just don't always know how I'm going to pay them. When the economy crashed back in 2008, I lost so much business that I practically had to live on credit cards for almost a year. And to this day I'm probably still paying on some of that debt. So, before you quit your day job and decide to become a personal trainer know all the pitfalls first. As difficult as it can be at times, I have no regrets in starting a personal training business. It has made me the person I am today, and I've met so many amazing people through what I do. All I can hope is that I've had a positive impact on some people's lives.

**Chapter Eleven**

**Silent Suffering**

The original title of my book was silent suffering. But I wanted a more positive title for what I've gone through in my life. Silent suffering seems kind of depressing so instead of making it the title of the book I just made it the title of a chapter and the subline of the book. I wanted to address suffering silently because I know I'm not alone in this. Just because I don't complain about it all the time or talk about it constantly doesn't mean I'm not in a certain amount of pain. I just found that people don't really want to hear about it all the time. Also, it's not in my nature to complain all the time or want sympathy. It's one of the main reasons that I talk to a therapist every week so I don't have to burden my family and friends with complaining about my pain. Most of us live with a certain amount of pain whether it be physical or emotional. When I was first diagnosed with ankylosing spondylitis, I told all my family and friends like I had some deadly disease. But at the time I really didn't know what the diagnosis meant. All I knew was that it was scary and I felt like I should tell everybody. After a while since I was mostly fine it didn't seem reasonable to talk about it all the time. I would have flareups that would result in a lot of pain but I didn't look like I had a disability so I stop talking about it. (It is important to note that just because someone looks fine on the outside doesn't mean something really bad is going on within, physically or mentally) I just decided to just get on with it. And at the time I could hide it. I think I did such a good job of hiding it that people forgot that I even had ankylosing spondylitis. It wasn't until I decided to write this book that I started talking more about it. When you tell people, you're writing a book they want to know what it's about so I decided to be honest about it which is surprised a lot of people. Only a handful of people in Los Angeles knew that I had this disease but since I didn't talk about it didn't seem to be a big deal. I got use to handling it myself and became silent. Even when I would tell somebody, they would just stare at me like I was lying.  There were many times that I wanted to scream out and vent about how much pain I was in but I never did. The only people I would really talk to about it is my therapist my best friend and now more recently my sister who has been diagnosed with the same thing. I found it very helpful to talk to someone that has the same disease as I do. When you talk about certain aspects of the disease and someone can relate with what you're going through you don't feel crazy. Because at first, I would question if this is all in my head or if everyone felt pain constantly in the spine. I questioned it because after several months of trying to find what is wrong with me a doctor suggested that it all might be in my head. I think a lot of times when they can't figure out what it is, they go immediately to "it's all in your head". It feels real but how would I know the difference between real pain or pain that was all in my head. Getting diagnosed was sort of a relieve. At least I'm not crazy. But when my sister was diagnosed a few years ago I could ask her about things I have experienced and the fact that she had experienced them too, let's me know that this wasn't just in my head. It was validation that what was happening was really happening. But it's important to know that my sister and I don't only talk about our disease. I think it's important not to let it dominate our conversations once we had discussed things thoroughly. Because sometimes focusing on it too much can be detrimental to your happiness. And I think if there's anything that I've done correctly is to not let it be all consuming. I don't feel sorry for myself and I never ask "why me?" And to this day I really don't know why I haven't asked "why me" but I don't think it would be helpful to ask the question. On a rare occasion when I'm in excruciating pain I do feel a little sorry for myself. I think to myself that it's not fair but after acknowledging that it's not fair I still have to decide to go on. Because as much as I yell at the sky that it's not fair, it's not going to change anything. All I can control is how I react to it. And I think that goes for anything in life. We can't always control what happens to us but we can control how we respond to what happened. I've always tried to take it in stride and I will have some good days and some bad days. I just try to have more good days than bad days. There are some days that I just have to give in and take the day and rest and do what I need to do in order to feel better. And then there are other days where I push through regardless of how I feel. One of my favorite quotes from any movie is from "Shawshank Redemption", "get busy living or get busy dying". I think about that quote all the time because as simple as it is, it is extremely profound. Because at the root of it; in life those are the two choices. In some ways when you have any disease or cancer you have a different appreciation of things. For me when I have a day of very little pain is it an extraordinary day. Mainly because they don't happen very often but when they do I have an appreciation for how things are supposed to feel. I think back of my time in high school I was in pain all the time. In a weird way, I kind of thought it was normal. If I said something, I was told by adults and doctors that it was growing pains. That was an easy fix-all for everything. Since I was told that it was growing pains and everyone had them how was I supposed to know any difference. I'm not blaming the adults around me, how were they supposed to know.

When you play football in high school all the guys had certain aches and pains so it seemed normal. I realize later that my pain threshold was higher than others. I find it funny that most people believe they have a high pain threshold. But how are we expected to know when you can't literally feel someone else's pain in less you experience the exact same thing. Now when someone tells me that it hurts to get a shot that tells me that they don't have a high pain threshold. I recently went to the dermatologist and he had to laser some things on my face and he commented that he didn't understand why I didn't flinch. I told the doctor that I recognize that it hurt but I could take it in stride. For me it ranked very low on the pain threshold. And maybe one reason is that I knew that the pain was temporary. He would spend 10 to 20 seconds on a certain location with the laser. It was intense but I knew it wouldn't last long. I have had flareups that have lasted 6 to 8 weeks where there is no relief from extreme pain 24 hours a day seven days a week. I'm not telling you this to feel sorry for me, I'm just trying to describe what I go through in order to bring a better understanding of people who are suffering silently. Most of us silent sufferers don't want to be that person that their friends and family avoid because all they talk about is their pain. I've always been hyperaware of that and that's probably why I didn't speak about my disease for a very long time. But I realize it's okay to talk about it as long as I don't harp on it. Talking about your pain doesn't make it go away but it does put a voice to it and sometimes it just helps to get it out. It is a fine line to talk about something and not overwhelm people with it. But I think I've done a pretty good job in my life of finding the balance. I also think that the older I'm getting the harder it is for me to hide what's going on in my body. It's getting harder for me to get out of the chair without looking like an old man and audibly gasp as I get up. There are days that my hips are so bad that it's hard to walk normally. Most the time it's just the first few steps and then I can get back to walking normally. That's mainly from the stiffness from being in a seated or lying down position. I have trouble sitting for too long are standing for too long or lying down for too long. I have notice in myself that I fidget in my seat more than I used to, mainly from being uncomfortable from the pain.

All that being said what is the answer. Well, there isn't an answer. I guess one answer might be to be kind to everybody that you meet because you really don't know what they're going through. When someone is short or mean they could be in a lot of physical or emotional pain and that's how it manifests within them. I have caught myself being short sometimes and easy to anger based on the amount of pain I'm in. It is rare for me but it has happened. I try to mentally detach from the pain almost like it's happening to someone else. Maybe like I'm floating above my body, that is sometimes the only way I can really deal. And as I sit here and write these words, I realize that I've been seated for a very long time and I have to get up. I'm realizing that I'm getting very stiff in my back and very uncomfortable and I'm starting to fidget. It looks like I can write about five pages before I have to get up. And I just have to accept that that's how things are and that it could take me forever to write this book. I get down all the time because I feel like I can never be as productive as I would like. I think part of the silent suffering is from the extreme fatigue. People with chronic conditions don't talk about the fatigue aspects of their disease. It's sometimes the worse part about it. It's hard to describe to someone that doesn't experience it but I think the best way of describing it is like having the flu. Most people have experienced the flu or something like it. Having a chronic condition is like having a really bad flu that puts you in bed for at least a week. Once you feel better you think everything is fine until you take a shower and then you have to lie back down for an hour because you are wiped out. It's kind of like that but it's all the time and with a lot of pain. Fortunately, for me the extreme fatigue only happens when I'm in a flare-up. The other times when I'm not flared, I still need a lot of sleep. Eight to nine hours. I don't always get that but that is optimal for me. Sometimes I get six or seven with an hour nap during the day. For some reason our society has made getting a lot of sleep a bad thing. That you are lazy or a loser.  And because of that I tried for years to push myself and only get six hours a night. I was constantly tired, falling asleep while driving, feeling crappy all the time, and very irritable. I had no energy to workout, drank too much caffeine to stay awake, ate too much to try to get energy, and overall, not in great shape (and I'm a personal trainer) Because I had clients at 5:30 am all the way until 8:30 pm it was hard to get eight hours a night. For the longest time I would get five or six hours of sleep at night and one- or two-hour naps in the afternoon and sometimes no nap. I would work on Saturday morning by eight or nine, so I only had Sundays were I could sleep in and most the time I would sleep until noon. It didn't "catch me up for the week" like some people believe but at least one night a week I would get ample sleep. I use to read about super successful people only get four or five hours of sleep a night and that's why they are successful because they didn't spend their life in bed. They would say, "I'll sleep when I'm dead". Which is funny, because studies have shown that people that get at least eight hours of sleep live longer. Or can live longer if you don't get hit by a bus or something. It's really simple when you think about it. The body does most of its repairs at night when you sleep. If you don't sleep enough it takes longer to get over something like a cold or injury. Over the last several years since I have gotten eight hours regularly, I have never done better. I noticed my productivity has gone up, my brain is clearer most of the time, and I have a lot more energy. I'm calmer and don't have as much anxiety. The benefits have been great. It doesn't make my disease go away but it makes it easier to handle. It is important to point out that it needs to be a good eight hours not an off and on eight hours. If you have sleep apnea then you must do something about it. It can and will cut your life short. Guys that I know that started to use a c-pap machine says its life changing. There are a lot of reasons someone doesn't want to use the machine because it's uncomfortable, loud, and takes a lot of cleaning and care. But it's worth it if you feel so much better. Now they have different things for sleep apnea that less evasive than a c-pap. If you have trouble sleeping there are so many resources out there to help. Maybe prescription, maybe a tea or meditation technique. There is help out there, you just have to want it. I know some of you are reading this and say well that is all good and well John but you don't have a wife and kids and a 60-hour work week and yes that is true. But if you can strive for eight hours a night, that's not a bad thing. It doesn't have to be perfect. Some days you will get only five or six but trust me you will be more productive in less time if you are rested. Imagine having a clear head during the day instead of always feeling hazy. There are going to be times in your life that no matter what you won't be able to get enough sleep. Parents of a new born might go a year or two without enough sleep but at some point, you will be able to if you remember how important it is for your health. If anything, I hope we can get away from thinking that eight hours of sleep at night is somehow bad because you're lazy. I love when I hear people say I can get by on four hours of sleep a night. Almost bragging as they nod off in their chair. If you fall asleep minutes after sitting down you aren't getting enough sleep, plain and simple. I know I use to be there early on when I started Frazier Fitness. My friends thought I was narcoleptic for the longest time. I would sit down and just pass out. I was working myself to death, thinking that's what I had to do. I think we all do that. But we should all stive for a work/ life balance. It's probably why Americans are in worse shape physically and mentally than any other country. We work all the time, we don't take enough vacation time, we are constantly stressed. Americans are number one in obesity, cancer and other illnesses. I think the Europeans' have it figured out. They work but it's not their focus. They close shops for two hours in the afternoon for lunch and a nap, and they holiday for a month every year. They travel and experience the world. Americans take five days, get on a cruise ship, lie around and eat and drink themselves into a comma. Not everybody but you get my point. We as a society need to do better towards a work/life balance. We need to stop putting poison in the soil, air, oceans, and our food. Yes, I said food. In the next chapter I'm going to go into details about our food. How bad it has become for us and how it can make our health worse or better based on our choices.

I never wanted to be that guy that says "eat gluten free" but you know what, there is something to it.

# Chapter Twelve

## Food

As long as I have been a personal trainer I've been into nutrition. And nutrition has changed over the years. Coffee is bad for; coffee is good for you. Wine is good for you; wine will kill you. Carbs are the enemy. And so on and so on. The truth is it's more complicated than that and simpler than that. I've learned that there is not just one way to eat. Everybody is different and everybody response to food differently. If you are diabetic you have to eat a certain way or you could die. There are diets for all kinds of conditions. For the longest time I didn't know that there are inflammatory foods. They are called nightshade vegetables; some are actually fruits. I know, I always thought that all vegetables were good for you. Nightshade includes: tomatoes, white potatoes, eggplant, okra, peppers and a few more. These vegetables have an alkaloid called solanine. While some alkaloids have positive effects on the body others can have negative effects. Solanine functions as an insecticide during growth of the plant. A natural insecticide to protect itself. Mainly, found in the skin and the seed of the vegetable. We don't usual think of a plant to be a living thing that tries to survive but that's exactly what it's doing. Now all that being said it does not mean that these are bad for you to eat. The levels of solanine in these vegetables are generally low and won't cause most people a problem. Everybody has heard the expression "too much of a good thing". Eating lots of these vegetables and taking in a lot of solanine can give you problems especially if the vegetable is not quite ripe. That's when the levels of solanine is high. If you have had a sudden case of diarrhea that could be from too much solanine. I'm not saying that everybody should stop eating these vegetables but if you have arthritis or inflammatory bowel disease or other auto-immune disease you might want to cut back or cut out these vegetables to see if it helps lower your inflammation. They are not the cause of the inflammation but may increase inflammation that is already there. For me, I would eat tomatoes for breakfast, lunch, and dinner. Always on sandwiches salads. I had no idea that could be making me worse. When I started Dr. Gundry's diet "The Plant Paradox" I was very strict. Cut out all nightshades and tried to follow his program as closely as I could. And I did amazing. It was very difficult to do but I felt better than I had ever felt. Several years later I'm still doing it but I'm not as strict so I'm not feeling as amazing but better if I didn't do it. I notice that I can do some nightshades but for the most part I try to stay away. On the Plant Paradox I can have tomatoes if I boil it in water for 30 seconds in order to remove the skin and then I cut it open and take the seeds out.

That's a lot of work so I don't eat tomatoes often. Moving on to other foods, there is always a debate about fruit. Is it good for you, is there too much sugar, certain fruits are good and some are bad? The way I see it no one ever got fat eating fruit in a balanced diet. That being said certain fruits can affect a diabetic's blood sugar, so for those individuals they may have to avoid certain fruits. Are you seeing a patten here? Everybody is different. What works for some people won't work for others. That's why there might be something to the Blood Type diet. I can't speak to that diet because I don't know much about it but if you are interested, it's easy enough to find out about it. Finding out what works for you could be some trial and error or you might get with a nutritionist that can design a diet that works with your certain situation. I found a low inflammation diet works best for me but maybe that's not for you. There is one diet out there that I think is harmful and that's any diet that makes you go into ketosis. Known as the Keto diet. It has had many incarnations over the years but it's usually the same thing, low to no carbs, high in protein and fats. The real problem is that the Keto diet works really well for weight loss and lowering blood sugars but it is a quick fix. I have had clients do it with my disapproval and every time it works really well and they lose lots of weight and they are so happy for a few months but eventually they have one carb and bam almost overnight they gain all the weight back and then some. I had one client that lost 40 lbs. on it and then gained it all back plus an additional 40 for good measure. And now studies are coming out that it could increase your risk for heart disease and other problems with internal organs. So, you see there is no quick fix. It's always going to be about a balanced diet and not stuffing our faces. Most people would lose weight just by cutting the amount of food they eat. Also, by eating smaller meals and eating more frequently we can avoid eating tons of food in one sitting where a lot of that will be stored as fat. A lot of times when we think we are hungry it's really are bodies way of telling us to drink water. The only problem is, we can't tell the difference between hunger pain and needing water pain. Next time you get hungry drink 16 ounces of water and the hunger pains will go away. The last thing we need to do, is eat slower. When we wait too long to eat, we become extremely hungry which makes us eat very quickly and eat way too much. When we eat very fast, we don't allow our brain to tell us we are full until it's too late. We ate so fast and so much that we don't stop until we are stuffed. Now, we have taken in way too many calories, sometimes more in one sitting than is recommended for the whole day. Once in a while we can't help it, things happened and we haven't eaten in 10 or 12 hours. That's fine but remember to eat slowly. It will keep you from overeating.

Now, on to meats. I have always been a meat eater. From the south you grow up eating meat and potatoes. And other stuff that is bad for you. In recent years, I have cut way down on meats especially red meat. I will have a steak once in a while and a burger once in a while but I try to have grass-fed beef. What I learned with my new way of eating (try to stay away from the word diet because it makes people do an eye roll) is that we eat what they eat. Although it makes since we really don't think about it. Taste good must be good for you. The main problem especially in the U.S. is having to mass produce our food. And I say in America because other countries don't produce their food like America does. Now on one hand we have an abundance of food. We throw away so much food we could literarily feed another country. With that abundance we have to compromise the quality. We stuff our cows with corn and soy to make them fat and juicy. This is not their normal diet and for humans we should not be eating huge amounts of corn and soy in our diet. Men should have very little soy because of the estragon like properties. You think you are eating meat but you are eating everything that humans put into that animal like steroids, hormones, and who knows what else. But I have noticed that grass-fed is more available in the stores and it's just a little more than the regular. But to eat out and eat health is way too expensive for most people. Remember when we eat out and eat cheap it's going to be the worse source for that food. For example: You go to a place, let's say it's not fast food but a sit-down restaurant and you pay $11.95 for a plate of chicken and a few sides. OK sounds healthy but in order for the restaurant to make a profit and keep their food price reasonable they are going to get the cheapest chicken they can and it will be full of all kinds of stuff. I don't blame them, how else are they going to stay open. This isn't always the case but the more expensive the food the healthier it will tend to be for you.

For chicken and eggs, I do pasture raised. Now pasture eggs are one or two dollars more than the regular eggs and that's an OK markup but pasture chicken is very expensive and hard to find. Pasture chicken are raised naturally, slowly, and eat what they use to eat, worms and the like. Not pumped full of corn and soy until they almost explode. I got a pasture chicken at Whole Foods, the only place I could find it, $20 for the whole chicken. And the whole chicken is small. Maybe ¾ the size of a Costco whole chicken that is $5. That is a huge difference not only in price but in the biggest bang for your buck. Let's face it, we naturally go with the cheapest option not the best option. Most of us have to budget and we can only spend so much on groceries because we have so many other bills to pay. For me I looked at it like this. I'll spend my money on healthier food and maybe spend less on medical bills and other things because I will be healthier. It's hard to know if it has worked out like that but I have spent more on food and I feel tons better and I have been healthier. I know I don't spend money on stuff for acid reflex anymore because my new eating has eliminated the acid reflex. I haven't had to go to the doctor as much. And maybe it will eliminate future medical bills, who knows. But I feel better and I think that's extremely important.

Last on the menu is fish. How can you go wrong with fish? Well, same as other meats, farm raised fish are feed corn and soy and that's not the best thing. Now I will once in a while eat farmed raised but not often. I try to mainly eat wild caught. And just like chicken it's the natural way and the more expensive way.

I'm not going to forget fast food. If you don't know by now that fast food is bad for you, I don't know what to tell you. But why is it so bad for you? Have you ever wondered why a Kobe beef burger at a nice restaurant is almost $20 and you can get two big macs at McDonald's for a $1.99? It might shock you to know that the food and drug administration (FDA) only requires the meat in fast food to be 35% beef. Wait, what? The burger you just ate is only 35% beef what is the other

65%? I'm glad you asked. The other 65% is what they call filler or pink slime. And what is that? Not to get too gross but it's all the left-over hooves, bones, eyes, whatever, you get the point. It's grouse, but everybody agrees it taste SOOO good. I don't eat fast food, haven't in years. Except on the rare occasion I've had In & Out because they have 100% beef burger. But this is something you will have to decide for yourself. You don't have to totally cut it out but at least cut down. I respect myself too much to eat that stuff.

On one hand we have figured out how to mass produce food at a reasonable price which is great. On the other hand, how we process our food is bad for our health. We are a feed society but we are a very sick society. We have more cancer, more birth defects, more autism, and more diseases than ever before. I can't quite prove it 100%, but I truly believe that what we put into our food, soil, air, and water is what is causing this. We put poison on our fruits and vegetables so they don't get destroyed by bugs but then we eat it. It doesn't kill us, at least not right away. We put pollutants in the air, and we dump deadly chemicals in our water, and we wonder why we are so sick. We poison the water that poison the fish that we eat. And all this could and should change but money and greed are the prevailing thing in our world. It would be nice if people cared more about doing the right thing than making tons and tons of money. There is a way that we can do both we just have to want to do the right thing. I've always said, "doing the right thing is always the hardest thing." It is so much easier when the cashier gives you too much change to just keep it. Or if you see a phone on the ground, it would be so much easier to just pick it up and keep it instead of trying to get it back to its owner. I always thing about it from the point of view if I had lost my phone and how much I would want it back. I definitely believe in karma.

So, when it comes to food let's all try to do the right thing.

# Chapter Thirteen

## Exercise & Recovery

Exercise, working out, strength training. It has many names and many forms. Weightlifting, aerobics, hiking, biking, boxing, yoga, Pilates, Swimming and so on. But what is the definition of exercise: Activity requiring physical effort, carried out to sustain or improve health and fitness. That pretty much sums it up. Straight forward and easy to understand but very hard to execute. You were probably thinking since I'm a personal trainer I'm going to give you all the tips and how to best exercise. Well, I'm not. It's not that kind of book. There are millions of fitness books that are going to tell you that this is the only method that works. If you do these things that I have done then you will be shredded in no time and blah, blah, blah. I'm not going to tell you that because it's not true. If I have learned anything over the years is "not one size fits all". For an example, if I tell a client that they have to run on a treadmill every day for 30 minutes to get results and that person hates running what do you think will happen. They will try it for a while, a week or two, maybe get some results but they hate it so much they stop, lose any results they got, and probably gain more weight because they felt like they failed. I have always been a trainer that has tried to find out what makes people motivated to exercise. What will they enjoy doing or at least not hate?

I have had the fortune to work with some famous people in my career. One of them was Steven Segal. They had tried with many trainers and none of them worked out. I knew on my way there, why all the trainers failed. It was kind of simple. They all tried to bend him to their will. When working with famous people especially those known in the movies for being an expert fighter you are not going to bend them to their will. I only asked a few questions. What is your goal, do you have any injuries, and what cardio do you like to do? He said sparring and I said OK, and I got the job and I started the next day. The point is, find that thing that you like to do or will tolerate and mostly do that. Some like to swim; some like to hike. I think the more things you try and the more things you like the better off you will be. Varity is key, mainly so you don't get bored or burned out. I like hiking but not every day. But there is one thing that we all should do even if we don't like it and that is strength training. Years ago, I started calling it strength training because weightlifting comes with some baggage. Weightlifting infers the more weight you lift the more fit you are. Also, I have had some female clients have a problem with that because it makes them think of big muscles and that's not what they want. So, I go with strength training because that's what it is. You start where you are, and you get a little stronger every day. And at some point, you might want to just maintain where you are. All I did during the pandemic is try to maintain where I was strength wise. I actually lost weight during the pandemic. Yes, I was one of only ten people that did that. Most people gained weight which is understandable. And then some people swung for the fences and gained a massive amount of weight. Most people said it was at of boredom, but I think some of it was anxiety and comfort. I'm lucky I guess I never get bored. I always have something I want to do like writing, painting, exercise, and yes watching a lot of TV. I guess as an actor it makes since I like TV and movies. I started to get into documentaries during the pandemic, mainly because I had the time. I always find it strange when I meet an actor and they say they don't watch TV. It makes no sense to me unless you are in New York and only do theatre and only want to do theatre. But I've met several actors in Los Angeles that don't watch TV and guess what, they didn't last long. Anyway, I digress. The point is it's important to do some kind of strength training. It could be the normal machines, dumbbells, and barbells, Polites, yoga, or log lifting, ditch digging and stuff like that. It doesn't matter what it is as long as you do something on a regular basics. And it can also be a combination of different things like cardio exercise. Most people are reading this and just want me to just tell them the secret to getting fit. The secret to getting fit is…. there is no secret. You see, it's individual. It varies depending on what you want to do. The more extreme the goal the more extreme the workout. Also, everybody has a different starting point. If you have never exercise in your life and you are 50 years old that is a very different starting place than an X college athlete that has just gotten a little out of shape. The thing that most trainers do with their clients and people working out by themselves is too much too soon. I don't care which one you are in the example above you still need to ease into it. Now someone with a fitness background is going to progress faster than someone that doesn't. But it doesn't matter. I have more problem with people that have been in shape than the ones that haven't.  Mainly because they have been in shape before, and they are less patient and tend to injured themselves. Out of the hundreds of people I have trained in 30 years not one has been the same. Now there are similarities and categories I could put clients in and I'm betting you want me to tell you the categories. So here it goes. As you know there are different personalities that people have like a type A personality. Type A tend to be competitive, workaholics, and impatient. Working with this type of person can be fun because they are willing to do what it takes; they are very focus and goal oriented. The downside is they tend to over train and can get injured, a lot. I don't believe that we are all one type, and we can never change. Most people are not just one thing. I've worked with type A clients and have gotten them to slow down and not over train and to meditate and to find balance in their life. I had one client, let's call him John because that's his name. Wall street type of guy. Living in Texas so up early to work before the markets open. I think he would get up at 4:30 a.m. and work until 3:00 p.m. pick up his five kids from school bring them to the club and train with me for an hour and then go home help the kids with homework or run them to their activities and be up until midnight and do it all over again. John was one the nicest guys I've ever met. He is that guy who would give you the shirt off his back. He also was very involved with his church. I had no idea how he did it all. But I know the toll it took on him. He would workout hard, throw himself into it with minimal results. Sometimes while working out between sets, he would nod off. Yes, really just fall asleep. One time I just let him sleep for like 15 minutes until his snoring woke him up. He also had sleep apnea and was quite a bit overweight. As nice as he was, he could be moody and depressed. It's no wonder, he literally was killing himself.

Results were slow and minor. You see if you don't sleep your body can not repair itself. As hard as he worked out, he should have been very fit. It was real evidence how important sleep is for recovery and growth. I worked with him for many years and can't remember exactly how we stopped. I believe it was because he moved. I did hear from him after he moved to Colorado. At some point he couldn't take the high stress, time consuming job and quit. I believe him and his wife started a religious camp for kids. That became their full-time job on a range somewhere in Colorado. I was never happier losing a client because he was finally putting his health first. If I've learned anything over the last 30 years is balance. That is the key to be fit, healthy, and happy. Being super fit is great and all but if you spend all your time in the gym, you kind of miss out on life. I know because in my early 20's I spent my life in the gym. Now most of it was work but there was several years there were I would start around 8 a.m. train clients until noon. Eat then workout for 2-3 hours then start training clients until 8 p.m. Things changed when I started training clients in other gyms and in their homes all over town. That's when I was lucky to get an hour a day or every other day. Since I don't have kids, I have always been amazed by parents that can still find time to stay in shape. I've seen people incorporate their kids with workout. They do push-ups with kids on their back, Squats with kids on their shoulders, and bench press their children. I think it's great because the kids love it, and you are teaching them good habits to take with them their whole life. I know it's not easy and it's not going to be perfect. I have found the older I get the less I want to workout. In fact, I can't remember the last time I was excited and really wanted to work out. I do it, but it's not as enjoyable as it used to be because it's painful no matter what I do. It started about five years ago. Before that if I was sore or tight or in pain, working out actually helped and made me feel a little better. But for some reason it started to make me feel worse. On the really bad days I'm afraid to work out because I think I could really hurt myself. I've really hurt myself just bending over. It's very sad and hard for me to accept the new reality I face. I really want to get back to that fitness level I was at in my thirties, heck I'll take four or five years ago when I trained a few times at one of the American Ninja Warrior gyms. I wasn't great at it, but I could at least do some of it. I feel like I'm fighting an uphill battle that I can't win. Every week feels like I'm starting over. I'll work out on Monday feeling good and the next day I can hardly move, so I'm scared to work out because it feels like I could just break. What complicates that is if I get hurt, I can't work and if I can't work, I don't get paid. Sometimes I might be erroring too much on the side of caution, which makes it hard to be consistent.  I tell my clients all the time that you will only get results if you can be consistent, and I can't even do that myself. It is the A.S. not being lazy, but still it sucks. Sometimes I only have so much energy and I feel like I must choose between working out or training my clients. A good example of this is during the pandemic I started to do yardwork and stuff around the property to off-set some of my rent. Since everything shut down, I lost most of my clients. I still had a couple but that was it. I had a deal with my landlord to pay half rent and work off the rest. It was a win/win, he needed the work done and I needed a way to off-set my expenses. Even with my A.S. I had to do yardwork which is probably the hardest thing for my back. That and sweeping and mopping. I would wait until I was having a "good back day" and would do the work on those good days with my back brace on, in the heat. It wasn't fun but I had to do it. I would limit it to two hours a day. One day I did just that and I over did it and couldn't train the two clients I did have that day. So sometimes I must choose between working out and work. It hasn't always been like that but for the past few years it has happened which lets me know that the disease is progressing no matter what I do. I wouldn't change anything; like the diet or the therapies or anything I've tried because I know if I weren't doing these things I could be in much worse shape. I know I've been talking a lot about how much pain I'm in and how it's getting worse but I'm really not trying for sympathy, I'm letting you know if I can do it so can you. It's not easy, it sucks sometimes, it's hard to stay consistent, but if you do a little each day you will be better off than you were the day before. Some of you might say "where do I begin?" It could be as easy as doing a few laps around the inside of your house. A walk around the block, one sit-up, some stretching. You don't have to do it all in one day and don't expect it to be perfect. I was jogging down the street one day and I guess I didn't realize how much I was limping, and someone pulled their car over and asked if I needed a ride. I think he thought that I injured myself and was trying to run to the hospital. Yes, it was a little embarrassing but a least I'm trying. And in life that's all we can really do is try our best.

As for exercise, do your best. Try. If you fail one day, get up and try again. If it's Friday and you realize you haven't worked out all week don't wait until Monday to try again, do something on Saturday. Everybody uses Monday as a reset day but when it comes to exercise every day is a new day. When I die, I think my tombstone should read "John tried really hard and never gave up." And that applies to everything that I do. I try to be the best trainer and massage therapist I can, I try to be the best actor I can, and I try to be in the best shape I can. In my mind I want to be in the best shape. I want to be one of the fittest people in the world and it's hard for me to realize I won't. But it doesn't stop me from trying. It has taken me 18 years in Los Angeles to get my acting career off the ground. I never gave up. I think that's really the heart of everything, is to never give up. Everybody that I knew when I first started acting in Los Angeles has given up. Now to be fair not everybody really loves acting like I do. They try it out and if it doesn't work out, they move on. That's totally fine. I didn't make a whimsical decision to give up a successful personal training business in Dallas and move to Los Angeles. It was very calculated and done with tons of thought. From as early as I can remember I have never given up on something I really wanted. If you want to get in shape, you will. I believe that you can do what you set your mind too. I know that's cheesy but true if you are 100% commented. Being commented doesn't mean it will be easy, it doesn't mean you won't have doubts, or you might have to change how you are going about it. For example, at some point more of my exercise will probably be in the water. If you keep your eye on the prize then you will get there.  And when it comes to fitness there is no there-there. I don't know any fit person that stops and says I'm the fittest I can be so I can stop. That's the thing about exercise if you stop you stop being in shape. You can cut back and maintain a certain fitness level. You can take a few weeks off but you can never stop or results go away. I see fitness like acting, you never reach the top of the mountain. You can always improve; you can always have new goals. As an actor you can win an Academy Award and still want new challenges, like theatre.

I watched the Olympics recently and you see these athletics winning gold medals and they ask them what's next and most of them say they want to come back to the Olympics and win another gold medal. There always seem to be more fitness goals out there. If you want to run a mile under 8 minutes and you achieve that, do you stop there? No, you probably want to see if you can do it under 7 minutes. Top athletes can only perform at an elite level for so long. Age is something you can't avoid. Some can do their sport longer than others but at some point, our bodies do tell us when it's over. Doesn't mean you can't do that sport anymore, just not at the level you once did.  I want to start playing basketball again. It's been a few years and probably five years since I played on a regular basis. Also, it's been four years since I tried America Ninja Warrior. I was never on the show, I just went to the training place a few times. I'm not in shape to do these activities right now. But I do believe I can do it again I just have to start. The biggest probably right now is the pandemic. It's been going on for a year and a half as I write this. In that time, I have tried to stay in shape but not going to the gym I'm just not as fit as I normally am. I do workout. I walk/jog, I have a Lifecycle, I have some weights and a punching bag but it's just not the same. I'm lucky I've stayed in shape. So many people gained a lot of weight during the pandemic. I actually lost a little. OK, don't hate me, here's what happened. I didn't leave my house hardly at all during many months of the pandemic. My big outing was going to the store once a week. I hardly picked up food at a restaurant. Mainly, I cook healthy, so when I went to the store, I didn't buy a bunch of crap. If you only have healthy stuff in the house, it makes it hard to eat crap. Also, my day started later so I would eat a late breakfast, a later lunch which became my main meal and a light dinner. I ate less than if I was busy and most importantly, I didn't eat out of boredom. I make sure that I keep myself occupied and entertained. I created a new routine and mostly keep with it. I made a to-do list and created a healthy routine of stretching, workout, and meditation that I still do. I did have huge gaps in the day where I watched way too much TV and Netflix, like we all did. I sleep 8-9 hours a night. (One upside of living by myself). I realized that I function best on consistent 8-9 hours of sleep. I know to a lot of you that sounds ridiculous but with an auto-immune disease that zaps your energy I have come to grips that I need more sleep than others. It's not that I can't go on less because a lot of my life I would only get between 5-7 hours a night. But I always felt like crap. I would fall asleep while driving. Any time, when I sat down, I would nod off. And generally felt terrible and was very irritably. For me ideally, I would sleep 8 hours at night and a one-hour nap in the afternoon. But since the pandemic

I've been able to get nine hours at night so no need for a nap in the afternoon.

What a lot of people don't know is that athletes like body builders sleep a lot. Nine to ten hours a night. As I mentioned, the body does the repairs while we sleep and that's when the muscle growth happens. Most people believe that the muscle grows while we workout mainly because the muscle gets bigger while pumping iron. But that is just increased blood flow to the area that gives it the appearance that it gets bigger. The working out actually tears down the muscle and the body repairs it at night when we sleep. You will not find a body builder that only sleeps 3-4 hours a night. I read a story of a body builder that got famous and started doing commercials and appearances and interviews, flying all over and his body building suffered. He had to cut back on the extra stuff and just get back to his routine. Most people don't know that body building is a full-time job. Eight to ten hours in the gym a day, very exact mealtimes, and nine to ten hours of sleep a night. That leaves very little time to do anything else. Or the same can be said about any pro athlete. I don't think most people realize how much time and effort it takes to be a professional athlete. Constant working out and constant recovery. Over the last several years more and more emphasis has been placed on recovery. It's been around a lot longer for athletes but it's starting to make its way into mainstream.

Recovery can be ice baths, cryotherapy, compression boots, e-stem, massage, and so on. The science has come a long way for athletes. Being a professional athlete has become very precise. From what to eat, to actually when to eat, to how much to train, when to train and for how long, to how much sleep, how the quality of that sleep is and meditation for the mind. It has become an exact science on how to be a top athlete. And just because we are not a top athlete doesn't mean we can't benefit and do some of what they do.

The number one thing we can do is ice an injury. Seems to be one of the hardest things for people to do. I have been told a million times by clients how much something hurts and they ask what should they do, they will do anything for the pain to go away. I tell them to put ice (or a gel pack or frozen peas) on whatever is hurting for about 20 minutes a few times a day. That brings the inflammation down. It's not going to totally cure you, but it will help in the process of healing. Most clients say absolutely and by the next time I see them 99% didn't do it. I usually get the answer, I forgot, or I didn't have time. And my response is it must not hurt that bad. Which the client gets mad and say it's excruciating. I believe if it was excruciating that they wouldn't forget, and they would make time. It's easy enough to do but well it sucks. It's uncomfortable and not fun. But a lot of life is uncomfortable and not fun, but we do it anyway. I don't like to ice unless the pain supersedes my normal threshold of pain. When someone use to go to physical therapy, they would always ice you at the end of the session. Unfortunately, they don't really do that anymore but instead they tell you to do it at home. I believe they use to do it at the physical therapist office because they knew that most people won't do it at home. But now insurance companies hardly cover the cost of physical therapy. We see it in professional athletes all the time. Sometimes icing during a game or taking ice baths after the game. It's a part of being a professional athlete. Unfortunately, we don't view it the same way because we aren't professional. But what if we did what they do. Maybe not at the same lengths as they do but if we emulate what the athletes do just a little bit maybe we can get some benefits as well.

I've discovered in more recent times, infrared saunas. It's like a dry sauna but with infrared light, which penetrates heat deep down. It's a great detox and I use the 30-minute session to meditate and stretch.

Stretching is one of the most important things we can do when we get older. When I was young, I could get up from lying on the floor and run as fast as I could and not hurt anything. Now I might pull three muscles just getting up. Sometimes I wake up injured, I call them sleep injuries. It's just a fact of life that we are less malleable as we get older.

Muscles tighten and joints stiffen. The best thing we can do to counter act the aging process is to stretch. I stretch everyday but you wouldn't know it. Massage therapists, chiropractors, doctors, all tell me to stretch. They don't realize that I stretch all the time but because of the A.S. I get tight again hours after I stretch. I don't even want to think about how stiff I would be if I didn't stretch. Or do all the things I do to treat my A.S. I know I would be much worse off and possibly get to a place where it might be too late to get some function back. So, no matter how bad it hurts I make myself be active, stretch, and do all the therapies I can to be the best that I can. The alternative could be so much worse.

For over 25 years I did everything I could to treat my A.S. holistically.  Chiropractic, massage, acupuncture, gluten free diet, stretching, meditation, and weight training. It all helped. I will never know how much, but I think I would be much worse off if I had not done everything I did. Despite everything that I did it ultimately didn't stop or cure my A.S. I do however think that it helped keep me in good shape. However, last year I took a turn. Kind of out of nowhere I got worse, a lot worse. My right hip started hurting beyond anything I had experienced before. I couldn't work out, it was hard to stand up straight, I was exhausted all the time. It was like I was in a flare-up all the time. I went from working out five to six times a week to one time or none. The pain put me over the edge. I don't think I realized how much being in excruciating pain effects my mental state of mind. I was having success in my acting career; in fact, I had the best year ever. But late in the year around September things really took a turn. I knew at this point that I couldn't live like this anymore. I made an appointment with my Rheumatologist and knew the next step was medication. It was inevitable that I was going to have to take something. I was a little upset that I couldn't do it all holistically but proud that I had put off medication for 25 years. Now I have to say that I have nothing against medication. I believe in western medicine, but I have always tried eastern medicine first. The main reason for this approach is that medications can have side effects and can become less affected over time. There are only a few medications for treating A.S. and have only been available for the last ten years or so. With the help of my doctor, I decided to try Humira. It has been out the longest so there is more information about it than any other medication. So far there are no known side effects for Humira. I was a little scared and a little excited. I think that the idea of having to inject myself twice a month for the rest of my life was my concern. But compared to having to have dialysis three times a week or having to inject insulin multiple times a day, I could get use to injecting myself twice a month. It took a minute, but it really isn't a big deal. Once I got my head around it, it's becoming somewhat normal. At this point I've had seven injections. After the first injection, I was shocked on how much better I got. Within three days I could tell a big difference. The pain was cut in half, I wasn't as stiff, I could move better, the psoriasis started to clear up, my energy got better and overall started to feel tons better. The weirdest part was times where I didn't feel any pain. Anyone that is in constant pain gets kind of use to feeling pain. It's not that you like it or that you aren't aware of the pain but you either just accept it and move on or you let it destroy you. When that pain is lifted it's very noticeable. It feels weird. I'm not used to being pain free, so it's an odd feeling and a little shocking. Don't get me wrong, it's incredibly wonderful, just odd. I woke up the other morning and laid in bed for 30 minutes feeling the lack of pain. I normally wake up and have to get up because it hurts to lay there. I just laid there enjoying the absent of pain. It's a feeling I can't describe. Is this what other people feel like? How wonderful. It's hard to have a bad day when you feel this good. I guess I never knew how bad things had gotten. And to say that there is a mind-body connection is an understatement. My mind is clearer, and I can get more done. I have so much more energy. I get eight hours of sleep and I wake up refreshed and ready to go. Before I could get 9 to 10 hours of sleep and feel exhausted and can barely get out of bed. I do question why I took so long to take something for my A.S. but I really wanted to do everything as holistically as I could. And I did. But I always knew that I would know when it would be time for meds and I did. At the end of the day, I don't regret how I handled it. Although things are so much better, it's not perfect. I do have pain, stiffness, some psoriasis, and I just had my first flare-up since I started taking Humira. It took a minute to realize I was in a flare-up. It started like it always does with diarrhea, then some hip pain, back stiffness, some fatigue, and some psoriasis. Most flare-ups in the last several years have been a 12 on a scale from 1-10. This flare-up I would give it a 4. It's not great but I can live with that for the rest of my life.

I can't tell anyone else what's right for them to do. This is what I did. But I would tell others that you should learn as much as you can about your condition. If it's medication you are thinking of taking learn everything you can about the different medications. Don't just rely on your doctor to tell you what to do. Learn everything you can and formulate questions to ask your doctor. Look into everything. Holistic medicine, western medicine, and everything in between. But I will warn you. Unfortunately, there are people out there that prey on people that are disparate to find answers. There are lots of snake oil salesman out there making all kind of claims that they can heal you. Over the years I have tried different things, some I would say helped a little and some that were total scams. Sometimes we think the more they charge the more it will work. It cost five thousand dollars because of all the rare ingredients. We had to extract the ingredient from a rare rock in the remote jungle in Africa, that's why it's so expensive. I would be very leery about a product like that. Always read what others say before you pay tons of money for potions. Sometimes some of these products do work, so just be aware and do your homework.

Although, Humira has helped me a lot, it does not make me 100% better. I still have pain and stiffness, some fatigue, some psoriasis but overall, it has help immensely. I really don't know what I would have done if I continued with the way I was going. I was quickly heading towards being permanently disabled. I think it's important to say that I don't just take a shoot twice a month and everything is fine. I still eat an anti-inflammatory diet, I work out and stretch, and I'm still careful not to do something that could screw my back up, like moving furniture.  I will always have to treat and take care of myself because I will always have A.S. unless there is a breakthrough in science and there is a cure. That would be great but in the meantime, I have to stay vigilant.

I finished this chapter quite awhile ago and things have changed a little for me. The Humira worked for me from December until September and then it abruptly just stopped. I thought maybe I got a bad dose or two. All the wonderful benefits felt gone overnight. The following months I got progressively worse. In late November something really bad happened. I remember doing the rowing machine at the gym for ten minutes. It was the first time I've tried the rowing machine in years. By the end of the ten minutes my upper back started hurting. This is not unusual because most the time I do anything physical my back will start hurting but most the time it goes away later. But not this time. In fact, it got worse and worse until I couldn't twist my upper torso. I went to the chiropractor which normally helps but this time it seemed to make it worse. I keep thinking it would get better or eventually go away like most flare-ups do but this felt different, like something more was going on. I thought about going to my rheumatologist, but I don't usually go to the doctor every time I have a flare-up. Since starting Humira I have to go to the doctor every three months to have my blood checked. I guess to make sure that the Humira isn't melting my insides. So believe it or not I waited until my three month check up to see the rheumatologist. Long story short, the small tip of bone on one of my vertebrae broke off. I'll never know exactly what happened. Was it the ten minutes on the rowing machine, perhaps. But the arthritis in the spine makes the vertebrae more fragile so maybe anything would have caused the bone to break. But now I have to decide the next steps on what to take. He gave me three options stay with the Humira and add another drug with it, start on a different drug or IV infusion for three hours once a week. I thought the easiest would be added something to what I'm already taking. Which is what I did. The problem with that is the drug is Methotrexate, which is basically a small dose of chemo in pill form. Not only that I also have to take folic acid pill six times a week and the methotrexate once a week. Great, exactly what I didn't want, taking two drugs which makes me have to take another because of the side effects. But what am I going to do? December was one of the most painful months (and that's really saying something) so I really don't have a choice if I want to be able to get around. Methotrexate has side effects, big side effects. And of course my first dose was when I went home for Christmas. When I go home, I am super busy visiting family and friends so I took the medicine in the morning and just went about my day. I was in one the worse flare-ups I have had so I was already really fatigued and not doing great. I made it through the day and went to my friend's house for dinner. I'm not feeling great but I've dealt with this most of my life so I'm putting on a good face but after dinner I felt like I was hit by a truck. I had to sit down and in about 15 minutes I needed to lay down. I knew that I couldn't drive back where I was staying. I felt terrible. I can't even describe how this felt. Maybe like I was coming out of my skin. Very nauseous, beyond anything I've felt before. Makes sense, it is a chemo pill. I had night terrors and sleep for 10 or 11 hours. My friend said I was screaming in the night, and I did wake up thinking that I was yelling out off and on all night. I felt really bad the next morning but once I got going I was OK by noon that next day. Since the first time I starting taking the methotrexate I decided to take it on Sundays because that is the only day I don't have work stuff. Every week since, the side effects have gotten a lot better. I'm mainly OK. If anything I feel a little off and a little fatigue. On the bright side the Humira with the methotrexate seems to be working. I feel tons better. Maybe not as good as when I first started Humira but what I deal with now is livable. My only worry is how long will this work. I know it won't last forever. At some point I will have to increase the methotrexate and eventually I will have to change to something else. I'm not going to lie, this sucks. I'm experiencing the very thing that I have been dreading. But now that I'm here I have to find acceptance somehow with my situation. I'm lucky in a lot of ways. I have insurance, doctors, medicine that I only have to pay $5 a month for, and access to therapies. If I was living in a third world country, I would have no help with this disease. I'm not rich but I have resources. I try in remember that others have it worse than I do. As I've said before, not to take away from what I go though or what you go though but just knowing that I have resources and support helps a little. Through the ups and downs I feel lucky anytime that I have some relief. It's not much but sometimes that's all I have to cling to and that will have to be enough for now.

# Chapter Fourteen

## Depression

Depression seems to be one of the hardest things to talk about. In the last few years, it is getting easier to talk about depression openly because of the push to rethink mental health. As much progress as we have made overall there still is a stigma with depression. The stigma of being weak or weak minded. Others will tell you to just "buck up", "get over it", "just decide to be happy", that's my favorite. I don't know anyone that decides to be depressed. I know from experience that nobody wants to be depressed but we just don't know how to get out of it. What most don't realize, is that there is a chemical component and hereditary component to depression.  And there are different types of depression. When a family member or friend dies, we are sad, and that sadness can turn into depression. That to me is situational depression. I've also experienced situational depression when I have had money issues which has happened many times over the years. My "situational depression" has turned into clinical depression. The definition of clinical depression is: A mental health disorder characterized by persistently depressed mood or loss of interest in activities, causing significant impairment in daily life. Possible causes include a combination of biological, psychological, and social sources of distress. The worse depression I've ever had was in 2010. I had been struggling ever since the economic collapse in 2008. I lost 60% of my personal training clients and was having trouble gaining that back. Like I have said before, personal training is not the most stable of jobs, especially in Los Angeles. I don't know exactly why the depression hit me then because I had been struggling for some time, but I know exactly the moment it hit me. I was doing my banking info and when I was done, I realized things were much worse than I thought and the shock of that hit me like a brick. I remember that I was so distraught I could hardly move. I had to leave the house to go train a client. I think I was on autopilot because I don't remember much of that day but I do remember having a hard time speaking. It was like I was mute. I went to say something and nothing would come out which makes it very hard to work out a client. I remember pointing at the exercise I wanted my client to do. My client obviously knew something was wrong but didn't really say anything. It was easily the worse session I have ever conducted, and I still feel bad about that till this day. Now, I would never have done that session but at the time I thought that my problem was money, and it would be stupid to turn down money. I did think about checking myself in somewhere but the next day I wasn't as bad. I was still depressed but I could talk. The only other time that happened was in December 2016 after I lost my lawsuit. Again, I was almost flat broke because I had almost taken the whole month off because of the lawsuit and I wasn't doing great because I was still dealing with fallout from the permanent nerve damage in my right foot that happened because of a botched surgery by James Wong, podiatrist. Yes, I'm using his real name so no one else has to go through what I had to go through.

When the verdict came down and I lost, I broke down in the courtroom. It was kind of embarrassing, but I guess everything that I had to go through for years was over and I had lost, on a lie. I was what they call despondent. I rushed out and got home and I realized I couldn't speak. My lawyer keep calling and I couldn't respond. I was near catatonic. I laid in my recliner for days staring at the TV.  I drank alcohol like you see in the movies, straight out of the bottle. Trash all around me. I had given up. I just laid there. I was days away from my trip back home to Dallas for Christmas. I knew that in the state I was in there was no way I could go. I cancelled. Blamed it on being sick, which wasn't really a lie because I was really, really sick, mentally. (Just a side note. I'm finding this very difficult to write. Now I know why I've been putting off writing this chapter.) I was doing two sessions with my therapist a week with daily check-ins. I didn't know what I was going to do but oddly I knew I wasn't going to hurt myself. Since I was going to be gone, I had nothing to do. I could have called clients and see if anybody wanted to workout but this time, I knew I needed to spend the next few weeks figuring things out. I don't remember much of those weeks, but I know every day I got a little better. I didn't see anybody; I didn't really talk to anybody except my therapist. After a few days I could talk again but I was spending more time away from people, so I didn't have the opportunity. I know I had to figure out what was going to come next. And at some point, during those awful weeks a phase popped into my mind. Are you going to let him win? Are you going to let James Wong decide how the rest of your life is going to go? I might have lost the lawsuit, but I was going to win life. And then things started to turn around. I'm not saying that one phase changed everything immediately, but it was the start of the recovery. I really did need to change how I was feeling, and that realization was the start. I still had months and months of recovery, but I knew I was going to make it. In therapy I said, "Rock bottom is a good launching pad." I don't know if I coined the phrase but if no one claims it, I will. As the new year started (2017) I got two new clients and that started me off in a better financial place and therefore started to help my mood. I built on it from there.  But I think this is a lesson that everybody can learn from. If you are depressed because of a break-up or losing your job or whatever it is, don't let them win, whoever they are. You are in control of how your story goes. That was a powerful lesson I learned from this terrible thing. I have built on that ever since. I started to engage with people more on the streets. I decided that I would say hi to people as I walked down the street. I smile all the time at people which has improved my mood. I try to be the light in the room instead of the dark cloud. This sounds easy but I put in tons of work to get to a better place. Happiness is now more my default than it's not. I really want to emphasize that this did not come over night. It was and still reminds hard work. It gets easier but I still have to work towards being happy, even when things aren't great.

Not only is there a stigma about mental health but also taking anti-depressants. I took them for years and they helped. I knew I didn't want to be on them forever, but I knew I needed them at the time. Like I said earlier, mental illness is also a chemical thing in your brain. If the doctor tells you that you have to take medicine for your heart, you do it. So why is it any different taking medicine for your brain? Because we are taught that taking anti-depressants is weak or whatever bullshit people say. Well, enough! Recognizing that something is wrong and then doing something about it, is one of the strongest things somebody can do. Anti-depressants work and they worked for me when I needed them. As I got better and better, I wanted to ween myself off the meds and see how I would do. If things got worse, I would go back on them. I weened myself off slowly with the help of my therapist and haven't had to take them in years. But if a day comes and I need to take them I will. I hope I don't, but I will if needed.

Other things I think has helped a lot is journaling, gratitude list, and meditation.

None of these things help instantly or one thing alone. I found that doing a lot of things help fight depression. I think the gratitude list and meditation helps the most. A gratitude list is a very easy thing to do. It's exacting how it sounds. You write down five things you are grateful for that day. Or just list five things in your head before you go off to sleep or when you first wake up. It can be anything. Or on the worse days it can be as simply as being grateful that you got out of bed. Or that I have a roof over my head. I especially like to do it before bed. Instead of worrying about things you have to do the next day you think about what you're grateful for and it makes it easier to go to sleep. There are no rules to it. You can be grateful for the same things each day, you can be grateful for five things, ten things or one. You can write it, think it, do it any time of day.

I really established a good habit during the pandemic to meditate every day. I've meditated my whole life but just off and on. The pandemic made me slow down and establish meditation to be a daily activity. Now I notice if I don't do it. Just like the gratitude list there are no rules. You can do it for a few minutes or an hour. You can do it seated or lying down. I found that when you take away all the "rules" it makes it easier to do it. I like a ten-minute meditation lying down. I use the Calm app on my phone. I also have longer meditations ranging from 20 minutes to 45 minutes and will do those occasionally. But my daily meditation is ten minutes on the Calm app. Also, I'll do it anytime during the day. Most people will say you have to do it in the morning when the sun rises and all that. Well, I don't get up when the sun rises so that would be torture to me. I do it when I have time. If we take away all the rules about these things it makes it easier to make it a habit. I found that meditation works well for me right after workout. I lie down meditate for ten minutes and then do ten minutes of stretching. I really like that habit, maybe you should try it.

Other things I found that helps with depression is helping other people. I have focused my efforts on helping the homeless. Most my depression has centered around money, or the lack of money to be exact. I don't have money to help the homeless, but I do have clothes and shoes that I don't wear and I go hand that out directly to the homeless. I do something that cost me nothing to help. Just my time. Every Sunday the gym that I trained at use to throw away all the water bottles that were left there that week. It's the reusable water bottles made of glass or stainless steel. I would pick them up from the gym wash them and fill them up and go hand them out to the homeless. Sometimes, they would be more appreciative of that than money. The point of helping others is to get out of your own head and go focus on someone else. We should help others because it's the right thing to do, but it's OK if a side benefit is that it helps you as well.

One time I was very down, and I went by a church during the day during the week when no service was going on. I was sitting in the pew very deep in though and this girl came in and lit a candle and started crying. I had to go see if I could help her in some way. I asked her what was wrong, and she went into the whole thing about her relationship and didn't know what to do. I mainly listened and then gave some good advice that seemed to be coming from somewhere else. This seemed to have a huge impact on her and really help her calm down. She looked at me with this amazed look on her face and I'll never forget what she asked. "Are you an angel?" I thought for a moment, "Am I?" and then quickly said no. She left and you know what, I felt better. Just by listening to her and seemingly helping her, it helped me. Maybe in some way we are "angels" for someone else. I think it's fine to feel better by helping others as long as it's not the only reason that you do it. I believe that when you go to help others you realize that you not alone in your struggle. Everybody struggles sometimes. But when we are depressed, we tend to isolate and think nobody else feels this way. There is a certain amount of shame associated with depression. I understand that because you don't want people to see you that way. We like people to see us in the best light possible. I've been so distraught that I don't even want my therapist to see me that way. It's human nature to hide what we perceive to be weakness. And there lies the problem. We perceive depression as a weakness, and we aren't supposed to show weakness. But what if we saw, not the depression, but the recognition of depression and taking action as strength. We need to look at it differently to change the perception. We view physical injury much differently than mental injury. If someone gets a broken leg, we tell them take it easy, take all the time you need to get better, you get disability until you can come back to work. But if we say we are having mental troubles you could lose your job. No sympathy no understanding, just judgement. There is a huge different in someone who is depressed and someone who is mentally ill. In all my depression I've never once thought about hurting anyone else. Unfortunately, some depressed people blame others and spiral out of control and try to hurt others. Once a person crosses over and thinks of hurting or killing others they have crossed over to mental illness, in my opinion. Since depression and mental illness is closely tied it makes it difficult to admit that you have depression. If you tell someone at work that you are depressed, they might think you are going to shoot up the place. So, we keep quiet. If everyone that has had depression wanted to kill people, I don't think there would be many people left. Not all killers are depressed. Some are and some are just really messed up. (Yes, that's the technical term.) We really need to take a hard look at these mental issues going on in the world today. Suicide is way up since the pandemic. With high inflation and things in the world seemingly out of control, there is a lot of hopelessness. I truly believe with love, kindness, and a little understanding we could do better and be better. If someone seems a little down just let them know that you're there for them. That alone could save lives. If someone is on the street and you see them crying, stop and ask if you can do anything for them. That little act of kindness could have just saved their life. Even if they refuse your help or even if they are mean to you, you should still ask if they need help. People being mean or rude to you has nothing to do with you. It is the way the person's pain manifests. Kind of like a cornered animal.

Remember we don't always get the reaction we want when we try to help. I've heard people say well if you're going to be like that than I won't help. You don't help someone because you want them to be eternally grateful, you help them because it's the right thing to do. Not all my interactions with the homeless is pleasant. But I try and if they refuse my help then so be it. It is important to note that you need to be careful if you go out to help people. There are some crazy and scary people out there. If someone is punching at nothing and yelling, do not engage. They are detached from reality and most of us are not trained to handle that. If you are going to help the homeless it's probably best to bring one or two people with you.

Helping others is a great thing to help your own depression but it's not that simple. Helping others can put things in perspective and maybe make you realize you don't have it as bad as others, but it doesn't just fix things. For me it wasn't just one thing but a combination of a lot of things over time that helped. I didn't just wake up one day and go I'm no longer depressed. Even at my lowest, if I could do just one productive thing that day it would be enough. Like I said most of my depression is related to money or the lack there of. Instead of having five things on my to-do list, I would have one: get new business cards printed. Next day: make one phone call to an old client. And so on. It's like a ball rolling down hill, you have to build momentum. Suddenly, I'm doing two or three things a day toward getting more clients. "They" say working out helps depression, which is absolutely true. But what "they" don't tell you is how do I work out when I'm so depressed, I don't have the energy? What I did is the same approach, one thing. Maybe I would do ten push-ups that lead to twenty. Or I would walk around the block that led to walking a half mile or a mile. Then I would do one thing for my mental health. I would meditate for ten minutes or list five things I'm grateful for or I would journal. I also, wouldn't force it. If I didn't get a lot accomplished one day, I wouldn't get down on myself. I would simply try to do better the next day.

Every action I took allowed me to take another action and so on and so on.  Here comes the building analogy: pore a good foundation. That's the daily habits you establish. Then every floor you add is your career, then your personal relationships is another floor, your financial security is another and so on.

The other main reason for my depression over the years is of course: ankylosing spondylitis. In fact, it is listed as one of the side effects of A.S. For a long time, I never put the two things together. Now, it seems so obvious. But why? Throughout this book I've talked about the pain of A.S. but sometimes the fatigue is the worse part. Sometimes needing 12 hours of sleep and still wake up exhausted can be depressing. Not being able to go about my daily life normally, like everybody else can be depressing. There are days that I drag myself out of bed and make it to a client and then go straight home and right back to bed. Sleep a couple of hours and get up in time for another client then right back to bed. Sometimes this can go on for days or weeks. It's hard not to get depressed when that is going on. Being unproductive is very depressing to me. I just get the bare minimum done. I can't workout or really go anywhere.  I used to force myself to pretend that everything is OK and I would run myself into the ground. I would fall asleep if I sat down. And worse of all I would fall asleep driving. It was very dangerous and I was just lucky that I didn't have a huge wreck.

It was ingrained in me that you must work hard and sacrifice to get ahead. Sleeping a lot or taking a nap was being lazy. But once I started Frazier Fitness and was training clients at 5:30a.m. until 8:30p.m. I allowed myself to take an hour or two nap in the afternoon. Not all the time but most days. That helped a lot, but it wasn't until more recently that I started to sleep eight to nine hours at night, and that really seemed to help the most. Since I don't start early any more, I can get consistent sleep and I don't need a nap. I know that once you read eight to nine hours of sleep, you instantly said, "it must be nice". Well, I would trade with you my A.S. for six or seven hours of sleep any time. It's not that I love all that rest, it's that I need it. I do love that fact that I can get into the car and know I won't fall asleep. Although I have accepted the fact that I need more rest it still can get me down. I've been trying to give myself a break and not get so down on myself for needing rest. It has gotten easier to accept what I can't control. But that has come with understanding what exactly is going on in my body. I wish things were different for me but accepting it has led to less depression in my life.

## Chapter Fifteen

## All the Injuries

I don't know if everybody gets as many injuries as I have over the years. I haven't been a huge daredevil or had a death wish. Most of the injuries are sports related, some are accidents, and some issues are hereditary. So, here's the list in review:

Head slammed in car door, twice.

Almost cut off middle finger with lawn mower.

Tore every ligament and tendon in right wrist playing football in 8th grade.

Too many concussions in high school playing football.

Minor knee, neck and shoulder injury playing football.

Mononucleosis senior year in high school.

Tore hamstring running track senior year.

Separated shoulder in car accident.

Almost died of chlorine inhalation.

Tore every tendon and ligament in right ankle (5th degree sprain) playing basketball.

Slight tear in other hamstring.

Broke and dislocated many fingers and thumbs playing basketball over the years.

Lower back goes out due to A.S.

Having A.S.

Diverticulitis

C-Diff colitis

At less 5 food poisoning or Montezuma Revenge episodes.

Crushed lower left leg in motorcycle accident.

Separated shoulder and cracked ribs.

Bruised, cracked or broken ribs four times.

Damaged nerves in foot from a bad surgery.

Some kind of skin rash (probably psoriasis from the A.S.)

Ten emergency room visits but only keep overnight twice.

Plantar Fasciitis.

That's all I can come up with for now. Seems like a lot.

But the top 5 are:

5. Torn hamstring in high school.

4. Nerve damage in foot

3. Tore everything in my ankle.

2. Crushed lower leg.

1. A.S.

Of course, A.S. is number one. It causes the most pain over the longest period of time. But the sickest I've ever been, was with C-Diff colitis and Diverticulitis. To date I've had ten rounds with Diverticulitis. And as bad as that is, C-Diff colitis put me in the hospital in quarantine for three days and took three weeks to recover. A.S. is number one because so many of the other injuries happened in part that I have A.S. My tight muscles in my back led to tight hamstrings that led to tearing my hamstring. Plantar Fasciitis is a side effect of A.S., so is psoriasis, and intestinal issues which is almost all my issues. I guess this is where I'm supposed to pull out an inspirational quote like "what doesn't kill you, makes you stronger". I think "what doesn't kill you, makes you wish you were dead, sometimes." That is a joke, but I do remember sometimes the pain would be so much that I would wish I would just die, if the pain didn't stop.

Most people would constantly ask "why me?" I know it sounds weird, but I've never really asked that. For one, it doesn't really help. And for another I know that I can't do anything when it comes to heredity. The saying "God gives His hardest battles to His strongest soldiers." Might apply. But I've always looked at it as it's not what happens to you but how you handle it. I'm from the "rub some dirt on it" generation. Suck it up "they" would always say. All that is good but sometimes it's good to listen to your body and not just ignore it. Sometimes some of that toughness can make it worse. I now don't always try to tough it out. I listen to my body and adjust accordingly. If I'm flared up one day I won't workout. If I need more sleep, I'll sleep more. By taking care of myself I've gotten better, despite the progression of the disease.

The other thing I did early on is not always talk about it. I did at first but after a while there is not much to say other than I'm in constant pain. Guess what? Most people don't want to constantly hear about it, especially when there is nothing that can be done about it. Many of my friends will be surprised when they read this book. Not my closest friends because I do talk more openly about A.S. especially in later years. Early on I think I was ashamed or felt like I was broken. I once thought having A.S. is a weakness but it is truly a strength, or at lease how I handle it is a strength. It would be nice not to have a disease. I think of all the time waisted sleeping or resting because I was having a flare up. I have cancelled many outings with friends because I just couldn't do it. I think about the many training sessions I had to cancel and work I have had to turn down because of A.S. At this point you probably think I'm going to say if I had a do-over I wouldn't change a thing because it's made me who I am. The hell with that! I would love to have a do-over and not have A.S. but that's not how it works. I guess I played the hand I was dealt and have done the best I could do. I do wonder if my life would have been deferent, it would have been less painful that's for sure. But would I have been able to help the people I've helped if I hadn't had A.S.? I can relate to clients like no other trainer. It's a struggle for me to stay in shape. Especially now. And as I'm writing this I really don't know if I will be able to get into the shape, I use to be in. The one thing that has changed in the last three or four years is that working out actually hurts my spine and makes me worse. I'm not talking about heavy workouts. Just about any kind of work out hurts me. Walking at a medium pace on the treadmill is O.K., anything else can really do a number. If I'm in a flare up I don't even, try to workout. I feel like the slightest wrong move will really make things worse. Stretching is about the only thing I can do. I can go for a few weeks before I can workout. So, the last few years I feel like I start and then stop and then have to start all over again. Most my life I worked out 5-6 days a week almost every week. It's been a hard adjustment and easy in some ways. I realize how easy it is to get out of the habit of exercising. Especially when it hurts to do it. And I'm not talking about the slight burning in the muscles when you work out. I'm talking about real pain. But I'm trying and I think that's all we can really do. The one thing I do, is make sure that when I don't work out it's because I'm really experiencing pain, not just being lazy.

The last thing I want to talk about (sort of) or I think is important to talk about is the one thing that happens with A.S. that defies any logic or explanation. I just found out from my doctor that this is related to A.S. I kind of always thought it was but never had any proof. I don't even know what to call it. The closest thing I can think of is hypothermia. It started in my 20's and only happened a few times. As I got older it happened more often like six times a year. Over the years and as the A.S. progressed, it started to happen more frequently, to maybe six times a month, to several times a week. I guess the best way to describe it as catching a chill. But that doesn't do it justice. One of the first times was getting out of a hot tub and having the cold air hit me. I got a chill and started to shake, violently. It was tame in comparison to now. It does seem to have something to do with going from hot to cold. Although it doesn't have to be cold, just cool. Mostly happens at night and mainly when I'm going to bed. I still don't understand it, but it happens more when I'm having a bad flare-up. I sometimes feel it coming on and can bundle up and keep it from happening but most the time when I feel it coming on it's too late. When it happens, I have a few minutes to get to bed and bundle up or it gets where I can't walk because of the violent shaking. I shake so bad that I feel my spine just aching and my internal organs shaking. My heart races and I'm breathing heavy. It sometimes feels like I'm going to have a heart attack. My skin is on fire, like all the heat is leaving my body.  I try to fight it. I take deep breaths hoping for it to stop. It does stop, eventually. I've never had the ability to time it. It seems to last from two minutes to ten minutes. On average I think it last three minutes but of course it feels like an eternity. It is extremely painful. But oddly I mostly worry about someone seeing me like that. It has only happened twice in front of someone and that was way back before they were as bad as they are now. I'm sure if someone saw me like that it would freak them out. I can't talk so I wouldn't be able to warn them. It feels terrible and I'm pretty sure it looks terrible. But the good news is since I started Humaira it happens much less frequently and I can live with that. It's so much better than it was. In high in site, I should have started Humaira two years earlier. These episodes are probably my biggest secret. Before writing this only my best friend and doctor knew about it. Mainly, because I don't know how to describe it. It is the easiest way to see I have a disease.

If someone were to see the episode, I'm afraid they would look at me differently. I'm sure it's not something you would forget.

Lastly, I've always wondered if A.S. is the reason that I'm still single. It probably has more to do with being an actor. I guess women don't like broke actors. Who knew? My deepest fear was realized a few years ago with my last girlfriend. I was going through a very difficult flare-up and needed to go to bed early because I was so exhausted. That made her mad and she said it. "I don't think you fight hard enough." Now I don't usually get mad but that really pissed me off! The amount of suffering I have dealt with most of my life, I feel like I have handled pretty well. And for someone I've been dating for eight months to say that to me was a real slap in the face. Obviously, she was not the one and I broke up with her not long after that. Oddly, I haven't dated much since. I do feel sometimes that I'm broken and who would want that. I do know it will take a very special woman to put up with what I have. Don't get me wrong I can still dress myself and tie my shoes, most days. I know having A.S. is a lot.

I recently dated a very nice woman who has M.S. We really bonded over our conditions. I think they call it trauma bonding. But at the end of the day, years down the road who is going to push who's wheelchair. I'm kidding sort of. I still have hope that I will meet the love of my life, just don't know why it's taking so long. I guess there is nothing left to say, so it's time to start wrapping it up. And now the last chapter.

## Chapter Sixteen

## The End is just the Beginning

Well, this is the last chapter, I think. When I started to write this book, I had no idea how hard it would be and how long it would take. I think it's been a year and a half to get this far. I look down and it says 198 pages. It feels like 898 pages. There were times when I was writing up a storm for an hour straight and I would look down and I only wrote four pages. Of course, I would go weeks and not write anything and then have to read what I wrote to remind myself and by the time I finished reading I had time to write one or two pages. When writing isn't your job, it's the last think that gets done. I have work, auditions, and all the other stuff in life. If I was getting paid to write, I think I would have finished a long time ago. My next book: I'll write two pages a day and I could be finished in around three months.

I think it's interesting that I'm writing the last chapter on a day when my back is hurting really badly. I did one hour of yardwork on Friday, and I've been crippled up for three days now. Not hard yardwork like chopping wood. Just pulling weeds, raking, sweeping, and trimming trees. Before I sat down to write I went to the chiropractor, took an Alieve, and a pain killer.  My back hurting this bad has put me in a bad mood and is just exhausting. But I decided to write about it while I'm going through it. Not sure if I have mentioned one of the most horrible things that happen when I'm in a flare-up but when things are really bad the nerves in my back are pinched and my right leg starts hurting. It is one of the worst pains from the A.S. that I go through. The best way to describe it, is it feels like my leg is in a vice and it's getting tightened and crushing my leg. On the rare occasion it will be in both legs and that's a fun few days. Since I've been on Humira, this is the first time I've felt the leg pain. The Humira has helped but not solved everything. I guess I got my hopes up when I first started because I was feeling so good. Or at least feeling not so bad. The hardest thing for me right now is not being able to do the things I once could. Everybody can relate to this, well of a certain age. I had to give up the one thing that I loved so much, which is basketball. I don't jog much anymore and now any working out seems to bother me. Not sure what to do about it but like always I'm going to try to work around it.

I'm writing this paragraph almost a week later than the start of this chapter. I was experiencing a flare-up on Monday when I was writing, and it got a lot worse as the week went on.  I took a pain killer which I rarely do. Not because I like to suffer but because I don't like how it makes me feel and I really don't want to become dependent on them. I was writing this chapter when it kicked in and I got loopy and stop writing. Unfortunately, this has been a bad flare-up. The worse one I have had since I started Humira. I want to go through the week and try to describe what a flare-up does.  Tuesday starts and so does the fatigue. Even after sleeping 8 ½ hours, I woke up exhausted. I'm extremely stiff, mostly in the low back. And of course, the diarrhea starts, all day for four days. I have a headache and my vision is a little hazy. I take Advil for the headache, but it does nothing. In some ways I'm lucky that I don't have a lot of work this week. To be honest work has been slow all year. I only have one client on Tuesday and that is taping an actor's audition. I worked at my desk for a few hours before nodding off, so I lie down and the next thing you know two hours have passed. The rest of the day I basically do nothing. Wednesday starts about the same but I do feel a little better. Believe it or not I do go and workout (lightly of course) and then go train two of my clients. I'm not doing great, but I do well enough to hide it from my clients. Why hide it from my clients you might ask? Mainly because it's gotten hard to hide it anymore. My clients can see me struggle more often, so if I can hide it I will. I know that most people would say that it wouldn't affect how they see me but if you're a personal trainer or massage therapist and you are constantly struggling a client might think twice about using your service. I can't afford for my clients to quit for my benefit. I try not to complain about it because that can really get old. If I can't hide it, I acknowledge that I'm having a flare-up and move on. The A.S. is exhausting but putting on a good face can be equally exhausting. At the end of Wednesday, I was happy I got through the day and was hoping that I would start getting better every day after, but that was not to be. I woke up Thursday after 8 ½ hours of sleep, exhausted, confused, and with blurred vision. My headache had come back much worse this time and I felt like shit. The newer side effect is my skin. Only for the last few years has my skin been affected by the A.S. I was told by one doctor it is psoriasis and another doctor thinks it's something else. Either way it sucks. I have breakouts in my ear hole, yes you read that right, my ear holes. And I break out on my chest and right arm and the most painful place is booth armpits. I do have a topical cream that helps and thankfully it only lasts a few days.  Oddly, I'm so tired and listless that I don't have a lot of pain in my spine. In a weird way I feel kind of drugged. It's like my body released some chemical that relaxes me so much I can't do anything. There again I only had one actor coming in for a taping at 2:00. I do nothing all morning and get it together enough for my client's taping. She has no idea how out of it I am, and I can't believe I got it together enough to do my job. After that I feel into bed for two hours but got up to meet a friend to watch Thursday night football. In hindsight I should have stayed home. My vision was foggy, and I was really out of it. I was more out of it than Monday when I took a pain killer. I hadn't taken anything other than an Advil for the headache and it still didn't help. Friday I was clearer and feeling a little better which was great because I had an actor coming in for an audition taping and I had to give a massage. And yes, it hurt to give the massage. Not terrible but not great. I was happy it was Friday because it was time to take my Humira shot which hopefully will help. Saturday was much like Friday, but the diarrhea had stopped and I was feeling a little better. No headache or foggy vision, the skin is starting to clear up, but I had muscle spasms. The muscle spasms don't hurt but the muscle involuntarily contracts constantly, sometimes for hours and worse case for days. It can be my triceps or biceps or back or legs, this time it was my forearm and it only lasted for an hour. Even if I have a flare-up the Humira seems to have cut down the length of time I have it and the length of time for the muscle spasms, diarrhea, and a lot of the other symptoms. It's now Sunday and I'm doing better. Not fully back to normal but close. Close enough to maybe workout tomorrow. Depends on what tomorrow brings. Monday it seems I took a step back. Back was hurting a lot, enough for me to have a e-stim unit on all day. A e-stim unit is a device that sends electrical stimulation to the muscle to help relax it. I still tried to workout but all I could manage to do was 20 minutes on the recumbent bike and stretch. Neither helped at all. I then had a personal training client and a massage to give. This flare-up has put me in a terrible mood. Monday was the worse. I think because I thought I was getting better Sunday and it turns out that I wasn't. I think it's the disappointment of what I thought the Humira would do. I was feeling so good, I thought it would continue. Now that I've had a very bad flare-up, I realize no matter what I do I can't get better. Don't get me wrong the exercise, stretching, gluten free diet, the Humira have all helped. I guess on some level I thought that I could "get over" it or "cure it" or have it be a minor thing. I would have many good days in a row and think, well maybe it's gone. I know, just writing that sounds dumb. But I have had more good days in the last year than the two previous years. I know in some ways I am better, but the flare-ups seem worse somehow. My theory is that when someone is in constant pain let's say an eight out of ten, when you hit a ten it's just a little worse than what you were feeling. Since I started the Humira I would have days of 3-6 pain level, so when it hits a ten it feels so much worse. That's my theory and I'm sticking with it. But it makes since.

Now I'm at a point as to what to do. Since I was 27 (when I was diagnosed) I knew I was on a clock, so to speak. I knew the A.S. would get worse as I got older. The plan was to be a full-time actor by 40 because I knew I wouldn't be able to be a personal trainer and massage therapist forever. Now that I'm 53 it's getting very hard, and I'm amazed I'm still able to do it. I knew I would need lots of money for therapies, massages, a trainer to stretch me, a chef to cook the ideal diet, and a maid. Believe it or not sweeping, mopping, and household chores are the hardest thing on my back. I used to love to clean the house. I could make it spotless in two hours. Now, I clean the tub and then lie down for a while to let my back rest. It's not that I physically can't do it but it's my back that doesn't hold up. Not even my back brace really helps anymore. So instead of being a well worked actor making lots of money to take care of my condition, I'm a broke actor that can't even get personal training work anymore. I haven't gotten a new client all year. In 30 years, that has never happened. I keep thinking it's God's way of protecting me and that I will get more acting work. It's either that or I might have to go on disability. Something I really don't want to do. I'm limited on other part time work because there is a lot I can't do. Basically, physical labor is out and that's the easiest work I could get. Even delivering groceries wouldn't be good. So, what to do. For the first time, I have no idea. This is the reality for people with auto-immune conditions. I have always used my experiences to help others. To show that you can overcome or work around obstacles. I have been able to find a way thus far and I have no plans of giving up. But that doesn't mean that I don't want to give up occasionally. When I think about giving up, I really don't know what that means. If I gave up, I would become homeless and that wouldn't solve anything. Or if I went on disability and just laid around all day wouldn't solve anything. Or worse case giving up means checking out of this life. I'm not going to lie and say that never crossed my mind but thankfully not for a long time. But what I realized, it's not that I want to end my life, I just want the pain to end. And I think it is what everybody that has contemplated ending it, wants. Whether it be physical pain or emotional pain. You just want the pain to stop. I find myself saying a lot to myself, "This too shall pass." And every time it does. It might take a while, but it does pass. I've had break-ups that were heart-breaking and could take months or a year to get over, but I do. I've had finical troubles that have gone on for a few years, like I'm facing now but it got better. At least the ones before. I've had stretches where I've had a flare-up last 3-4 months, but they do eventually end. The saying "with age comes wisdom" is true. When I was young, I thought everything was the end of the world. A break-up in high school, "NO ONE WILL EVER LOVE ME AGAIN." Fast forward 20 years later, "I guess that wasn't the one, what did I learn from that." If enough time passes something will change. It's taken me 30 years before I was in a movie that people could watch on TV. Don't know why it took so long but it wouldn't have happened if I gave up. An important point here: I never stopped working towards the acting. I have talked to other actors that say well I took a year or two off. That works if you are a famous actor but if you are trying to build a career you can never "take time off" more than a vacation, maybe. And I believe that applies to my A.S. I can never stop trying to feel as good as I can. I know that lying around all the time will make me worse. I have to stretch no matter how painful; I have to workout no matter how hard it is to do, and I have to eat healthy to give myself a chance to fight the disease. I don't know what the future holds for me. I don't know how bad it will get. I don't know if I can pay the bills next month. I don't know if I'll be a full-time actor ever. But I do know I will never give up trying. And really that's all we can do in life, is not give up.

My words of wisdom: No matter what you face, rather it be physical or emotional or mental "Never stop fighting." Try everything you can to reach your goals. Never stop fighting whatever disease you have. Accept that it's going to be hard and not always go to plan. Know when to give yourself a break mentally or physically. Accept that there might be physical limitations. And remember you only lose if you give up. I want to close with a quote from a singer named Night Bird. She was on America's Got Talent in 2021 and had stage 5 cancer. She went on the show and sang a song she wrote called "It's OK". It's a wonderful song and very emotional. But when asked why she came on the show she simply said, "You can't wait until life isn't hard anymore, before you decide to be happy." What a quote to live by. She unfortunately died shortly after but her impact on the world will last forever. Seeing someone face a terminal disease with such courage and dignity is awe inspiring. Something we should all strive to be in this life.

The End......or to be continued.